DATE DUE

HIGHSMITH 45-220

Setting the Limit

SETTING THE LIMIT

Occupational Health Standards
and the Limits of Science

SVEN OVE HANSSON
Department of Philosophy
Uppsala University

New York   Oxford
OXFORD UNIVERSITY PRESS
1998

Oxford University Press

Oxford New York
Athens Auckland Bangkok Bogota Bombay
Buenos Aires Calcutta Cape Town Dar es Salaam
Delhi Florence Hong Kong Istanbul Karachi
Kuala Lumpur Madras Madrid Melbourne
Mexico City Nairobi Paris Singapore
Taipei Tokyo Toronto Warsaw

and associated companies in
Berlin Ibadan

Copyright © 1998 by Oxford University Press

Published by Oxford University Press, Inc.
198 Madison Avenue, New York, New York 10016

Oxford is a registered trademark of Oxford University Press

All rights reserved. No part of this publication may be reproduced,
stored in a retrieval system, or transmitted, in any form or by any means,
electronic, mechanical, photocopying, recording, or otherwise,
without the prior permission of Oxford University Press.

Library of Congress Cataloging-in-Publication Data
Hansson, Sven Ove, 1951-
Setting the limit :
occupational health standards and the limits of science /
Sven Ove Hansson.
p. cm.
Includes bibliographical references and index.
ISBN 0-19-512160-0
1. Threshold limit values (Industrial toxicology)
2. Industrial hygiene.
3. Industrial toxicology.
I. Title. RA1229.5.H36 1998 615.9'02—dc21 97-34725

9 8 7 6 5 4 3 2 1

Printed in the United States of America
on acid-free paper

PREFACE

Occupational exposure limits are a prime example of the interaction between science and values. In particular, there are few other policy areas in which the implications of epistemic uncertainty emerge more clearly. I have chosen this area for a detailed study, both for these theoretical reasons and because of its social importance.

As in so many other areas, we can come to grips with the philosophical issues only if we plunge deeply into the empirical sciences. Chapter 1 introduces the science of toxicology, with an emphasis on its epistemological aspects. The three chapters that follow analyze in depth three lists of occupational exposure limits and the documentation that has been developed to substantiate them. The threshold limit values of the American Conference of Governmental Industrial Hygienists (Chapter 2) have been selected because of their dominant role worldwide. The official German list (Chapter 3) is particularly interesting since it is claimed to be based exclusively on considerations of health. The offical Swedish list (Chapter 4) was chosen because it seems to contain the lowest exposure limits in the Western world.

In Chapter 5, proposals are put forward for new ways to organize exposure limits and to evaluate toxicological data for regulatory purposes. This chapter has three leading ideas: first, epistemic uncertainty, and not only known risks, should be taken into account and protected against; second, the unavoidable compromises between health and economics should be made openly, not hidden behind false claims of absolute safety or purely health-based regulations; and third, such compromises should be as limited in scope as possible, and thus refer to particular uses of a substance, rather than to all uses.

This research was supported by grants from the Swedish Council for Planning and Coordination of Research and the Swedish Council for Work Life Research, that are gratefully acknowledged. Thanks are due to Maria Lewander (Grön Idé) for her competent technical assistance, to the library staff of the National Institute for Working Life (Stockholm) for excellent services, to Mario Bunge and Barry Pless for encouragement and support, to Bo Holmberg, Johan Högberg, Per Lundberg, and Bengt Midgren for valuable comments on an earlier version of Chapter 4, and to Mikael Johannesson, Christina Rudén, and Mats Wingborg for many helpful discussions.

Uppsala   S.O.H.
June 1997

CONTENTS

1. Regulating the Unknown   1
   Clinical medicine and the science of health   1
   Science and occupational health   3
   Two types of error   7
   Epistemic asymmetry   11
   Exposure limits   12

2. The Most Influential Values   17
   The ACGIH and its TLVs   17
   Health-based, realistic, or both?   20
   Harmful effects below the TLVs   24
   The use of corporate information   27
   Unorthodox toxicology   29
   Conclusions   33

3. Purely Health-based Values? 35
In what sense health-based? 36
Irritation and worse 39
The protection of subpopulations 43
Protecting the unborn 45
Margins of safety and unsafety 47
Human effect levels 49
Animal no-effect levels 53
Animal effect levels 60
On not learning from experience 65
Standards of evidence 66
Questionable reporting 70
Conclusions 72

4. The Lowest Values 75
The development of Swedish exposure limits 75
The impact of consensus reports 78
Critical effects 81
Irritation effects 83
Respiratory diseases 88
Effects on the nervous system 91
Other nonmalignant critical effects 93
Cancer 96
The quality of no-effect levels 98
Conclusions 102

5. Setting Better Standards 103
An impossible task? 103
Health-based exposure limits 105
Levels of aggregation 106
A residual exposure limit 109
Interpretative conservativity 110

Statistical evaluations 113
The role of science in standard setting 119

Appendix: How to Compare Exposure Limits 123

Notes 133

Glossary 141

References 147

Index 157

1

REGULATING THE UNKNOWN

Toxicity depends on the dose. Therefore, human health can be protected in dangerous environments if there are well-founded exposure limits and compliance with them. This is the rationale for occupational exposure limits (OELs).[1] The purpose of this introductory chapter is to outline the nature of the scientific evidence available to standard setters as a background to the detailed study of the three standard-setting practices described in Chapters 2–4.

CLINICAL MEDICINE AND THE SCIENCE OF HEALTH

Occupational medicine is part of the science of human health. Despite its dominance in present-day medicine, the scientific approach to human health is of surprisingly late origin. Traditionally, treatments were based on a combination of theoretical doctrines and unsystematized experiences. Only in the nineteenth century did the pioneers of scientific medicine propose that the effectiveness of therapeutic methods should be subjected to scientific studies (Booth 1993).

The French physician Pierre Charles-Alexandre Louis (1787–1872) was one of these pioneers. He advocated a *numerical method*, consisting in the comparison of groups of patients who had received different treatments. In an epidemic situation when many patients were subject to the same condition, they could be randomly distributed between two kinds of treatment. From the differences between the two groups, the relative efficiency of the two treatments could then be evaluated (Wilkinson 1993).

One of the most important early applications of this numerical method was a study of the treatment of pneumonia reported in 1849 by the Austrian physician Joseph Dietl (1804–1878). He compared three groups of pneumonia patients.[2] One group, consisting of 85 patients, had been treated with bloodletting, which was at this time the almost universally prescribed therapy for pneumonia. Another group, with 106 patients, had received large doses of an emetic, which was the major competing therapy. A third group of 189 patients had received no specific treatment at all. The mortality in the first group was 20.4%, in the second group 20.7%, and in the third group 7.4% (Dietl 1849, esp. p. 122).

This result was a great embarrassment to the medical profession, but the new information was grudgingly accepted, and a couple of decades later bloodletting for pneumonia was condemned in all the major medical handbooks. Yet this study was an isolated episode, and it was only in the twentieth century that clinical tests became a standard procedure in medicine.

It is important to understand that physicians before the present age of clinical testing were as astute as their present-day colleagues. The example of pneumonia treatment shows that human cognitive powers are surprisingly weak with respect to stochastic events. Even a large effect such as the increased mortality that follows bloodletting will be missed unless data are collected and evaluated in a systematic, i.e., statistical way. Unsystematized practical experience is much less reliable than we would like to believe even if it is the experience of a trained practitioner. Scientific medicine has learned this lesson and has therefore adopted clinical tests as its touchstone of therapeutic efficacy.

SCIENCE AND OCCUPATIONAL HEALTH

Whereas the diagnosis and treatment of diseases is the predominant activity in most of clinical medicine, occupational medicine is focused much more on the search for cause–effect relationships between health impairment and occupational factors. Unfortunately, no scientific method is available for the latter task that is as reliable as clinical tests are for the evaluation of therapeutic methods. The closest method would be *experiments on humans* in which people are subjected to controlled exposures and their health is carefully monitored for possible effects. For both ethical and legal reasons, such experiments are normally not performed (Pfeiffer 1986, p. 262). Instead, two major roads to knowledge are available for the scientific study of occupational health hazards. One of them is *non-experimental observations on humans*. These normally take the form of epidemiological studies in which groups of people are compared statistically in the search for associations between disease incidence and environmental or other causal or explanatory factors. The other road to knowledge is *experiments on non-humans*, i.e., laboratory studies that make use of animals, bacteria, or tissue cultures. The scientist is (presumably) relieved of ethical responsibility, in the first case since she has not herself instigated the exposures, and in the second case since she uses animals rather than human beings.

The simplest form of observation on humans is the *case report*, commonly made by a physician who has observed signs of disease among persons exposed to a substance. Although many important toxicological discoveries originated in this way, case reports are often difficult to interpret. They are commonly seen as sources of ''hypotheses, which can then be tested by epidemiologists or laboratory scientists or both'' (Miller 1978, p. 118).

More solid knowledge about cause–effect relationships in occupational health comes primarily from epidemiological research. The effects of major health hazards on the workplace, such as asbestos, lead, and vinyl chloride, among many others, have been convincingly identified and quantified in epidemiological studies. Nevertheless, epidemiology has been unable to answer most of the questions for which occupational health practitioners need answers. Many epidemiological studies have proved inconclusive, largely due to the many factors that can influence the prevalence of disease in human populations. Epidemiology also suffers from the crucial disadvantage of being feasible only *post factum*. Typically, epidemiological studies can be performed only when hundreds of workers have been exposed to a substance for many years. Therefore, although epidemiology is indispensable, it has to be supplemented with study methods that are applicable prior to human exposure. This is where laboratory experiments on animals come in.

In such experiments, one or several animal groups are exposed to a potentially toxic substance. Their health status is compared to that of an unexposed control group that has received the same treatment—apart from the exposure—as the exposed animals. It has sometimes been questioned whether there is any valid basis for implying consequences for human health from the findings of animal experiments. If conclusions must be drawn with absolute certainty, then there is no basis for comparison. If, on the other hand, less than certain conclusions are accepted, then such studies have value.

The basis for their value is the high degree of biochemical similarity between humans and the more common experimental animals, such as rats, mice, guinea pigs, rabbits, and pigs. The major features of cell organization are the same. Most metabolic processes, including those involved in detoxification and bioactivation, are largely the same. For instance, a human liver cell and the liver cell of a rat are much more similar in structure and metabolism than, say, a human liver cell and a human kidney cell. In a large number of cases, toxic effects that have been observed in humans have also been replicated in animal experiments.

Although animal experimentation has predictive power, unfortunately the predictions are far from perfect. There are substances to which humans are much more, or much less, sensitive than the common laboratory animals. Differences in sensitivity are often due to differences in metabolism. Such differences can be found not only between species but also between individuals of the same species. In particular, they can be found in the human species. In addition to the genetic variability of the human race, factors such as nutrition, drinking habits, and smoking, among many others, may influence the metabolic fate of toxic substances.

The animal groups used in toxicological experiments belong to highly inbred strains. The homogeneity of animal groups is a basic feature not only in toxicology but in experimental biology in general. There are strong methodological reasons for this practice. With inbred strains, smaller animal groups are needed to obtain statistically reliable results. Furthermore, independent replication of experiments is greatly facilitated by the availability of animals that are virtually identical genetically to those used in the original experiment.

But whereas genetic and environmental homogeneity increases the reliability of animal experiments, it decreases their validity for the assessment of human toxicity. The difference between the variability of the human population and the nonvariability of laboratory animals can be just as important in species extrapolation as the difference between the average rat and the average human.

To some extent, the genetic homogeneity of laboratory strains can be compensated for by the use of several species and strains. For obvious reasons, a strain whose metabolism of a particular substance is similar to that in humans is of particular interest in studies of this substance. However, results of studies involving an animal strain with a metabolism that differs from the most common human metabolism may be relevant to some (unknown) human subpopulation with a deviant metabolic pattern. This was aptly pointed out by Gillette and Estabrook:

> It may well be that virtually any incidence of toxicity obtained with virtually any species or strain of animal may mimic that obtained with one

of the human subpopulations. Even contradictory results may be relevant to different subpopulations. It is prudent, therefore, to assume that qualitative results obtained in toxicity studies with any animal species are possibly relevant to some fraction of the human population. (1987, p. 358)

A further factor must be mentioned that complicates species extrapolation: Some health effects are specifically human or at least very difficult to discover in experimental animals. This is particularly true of functional disorders of the central nervous system. Disturbances in more subtle human intellectual or emotional abilities cannot in general be correlated with changes in animal behavior.

Besides using animals, toxicological experiments can be performed on cell cultures and bacteria. These tests are orders of magnitude less expensive than animal experiments, and ethically they are much less problematic. Their main drawback is that their interpretation requires a further type of extrapolation that is not needed in the interpretation of animal experiments, namely, what we may call *part-to-whole extrapolation*.

The human body consists of a large number of different cell types. Each of these cell types has specialized functions and unique metabolic properties. The interplay between different cell types makes all the difference between a human and an ameba. Therefore, it is only to be expected that some substances can be much more or much less toxic to an organism than to any isolated cell type from that organism. One mechanism by which a substance can be more toxic is bioactivation: It is chemically transformed in one type of cell into a new form that is much more injurious than the original substance to certain other cells. Indeed, some substances that are highly toxic to entire organisms do not appear to be toxic in tests on isolated cells or on subcellular systems (Ahlborg et al. 1988, p. 56).

Part-to-whole extrapolation can be done in a fairly reliable way in cases in which adequate *mechanistic knowledge* is available. If the mechanisms of a toxic action are known in detail, then it should be both possible and advantageous to study its crucial stages in small, isolated systems. To date, the best example is genotoxicity tests that make use of the high degree of similarity between DNA in lower organisms, including bacteria, and DNA in humans. The results of genotoxicity tests are related to carcinogenicity and to inherited disease, but the correlations are far from perfect (Zeiger 1987).

The modern approach to cause–effect relationships in occupational health, as outlined above, is of quite recent origin. The transition to the modern scientific paradigm took place still later in occupational medicine than in clinical medicine. Well after World War II, the dominant source of knowledge was practical clinical experience. Data on pathology in deceased workers were a much more important source of knowledge than data (including nonlethal effects) obtained from epidemiology. The use of epidemiological evidence of noninfectious disease was not fully accepted in the medical world until after the Surgeon General's first report on the health hazards of smoking in 1965 (Egilman 1992, p. 457; Morgan 1992, p. 437). New methods of animal experimentation developed since the 1960s have also had a strong influence on occupational medicine.

TWO TYPES OF ERROR

Two major types of error can be made when assessing the toxicity of a substance: ascribing to it toxic effects that it does not have or failing to ascribe to it toxic effects that it in fact has. These are the same two types of error that appear in all scientific disciplines: In the first case, you conclude that there is a phenomenon or an effect that in fact does not exist. This is called *type I error* (false positive). In the second case, you miss an existing phenomenon or effect. This is called *type II error* (false negative). In scientific practice, these types of error are very different. Type I errors are extremely serious. To make such an error means to draw an unwarranted conclusion, to believe something that should not be believed. Such errors lead us astray, and if too many of them are committed, then scientific progress will be blocked by pursuit down all sorts of blind alleys.

Type II errors are much less serious from a scientific point of view.

To make such an error means keeping an issue open instead of adopting a correct hypothesis. Of course, not everything can be kept open, and science must progress when there are reasonable grounds for doing so. Nevertheless, failing to proceed is a much less serious error than moving in the wrong direction. Isaac Levi even maintains that type II errors are not, properly speaking, errors (Levi 1962).

This difference in severity between the two types of error can also be expressed in terms of burden of proof. When determining whether or not a scientific hypothesis should be accepted for the time being, the onus of proof falls squarely on its adherents. Those who claim the existence of a still unproven effect—such as a toxic effect of a chemical substance—must prove their claim.

This is all very well so long as we stay in the realm of pure science. However, when results from science are applied in other areas, there may be good reasons for distributing the burden of proof differently. The application of toxicology to policy decisions is a clear example. There is no sensible ethical motivation for total neglect of type II errors in a regulatory context. To the contrary, most people consider it vital to avoid type II errors—at least when their own health is concerned. More concretely, we wish to protect ourselves against suspected health hazards even if the evidence is much weaker than that required for scientific proof (Rudner 1953; Jellinek 1981). Therefore, *any ethically defensible standard of the burden of proof for regulatory applications will have to differ significantly from the burden of proof that prevails in toxicology for purely scientific purposes.*

Since scientists are normally not trained in decision theory or in the philosophy of science, this has not always been well understood by toxicologists and epidemiologists. We sometimes find scientists unreflectingly applying intra-scientific standards of proof as criteria for when preventive measures should be taken. Since these criteria give absolute priority to avoiding type I errors over type II errors, the outcome may very well be that risks are taken that few of us would accept when the lives and health of our own families are at stake. *By applying standard scientific criteria out of context, a scientist can become an unwilling ally of policies that run counter to the interests of public health*. The history of occupational medicine is replete with examples of this, one of which was described by William Schultz:

> [I]t is helpful to recall the debates over the Color Additive Amendments of 1960. At the time, Eli Lilly & Co., the principal manufacturer of DES [diethylstilbestrol], opposed the Delaney Clause. One of its Vice Presidents, Dr Thomas Carney, argued that the basic assumption of the Delaney Clause, that animal carcinogens may cause cancer in humans, is incorrect. As an example, he used DES, which he pointed out had been found to cause cancer in more than one species of animals. Dr. Carney then observed that DES has been used in human drugs for more than 20 years and was so safe that doctors were prescribing it to thousands of women to prevent miscarriages. He then quoted experts who had concluded that DES was safe for humans and that any correlation between DES and human cancer was "most probably mythical."
>
> Twenty years later, with the benefit of hindsight, we are much wiser. We know that DES causes a rare form of vaginal and cervical cancer of daughters of the pregnant women who took the drug....
>
> Dr. Carney could not have known in 1960 what we know today because the first study demonstrating a link between DES and human cancer was not published until 1971. However, in the same way, we do not know as much today as our successors will know 20 years from now. (1988, pp. 525–526)

Two technical concepts used in toxicology are particularly problematic in connection with type II errors. One of these is *statistical significance*, which is used throughout science as a measure of the risk of type I errors. An effect (such as toxicity) has been shown with statistical significance (at the critical level 0.05) in a particular study if the probability of the results obtained would be less than 0.05 if no effect (here, no toxicity) existed. It is usually considered a necessary (but not sufficient) precaution against type I errors to regard results as inconclusive if they are not statistically significant.

Significance testing can be seen as a mathematical expression of the conventional burden-of-proof standard in science that gives absolute precedence to avoiding type I errors over type II errors. Nevertheless, the dividing line between significance and nonsignificance has in practice often also been used as a dividing line between the decision that "the regulatory body should act as if an effect has been demonstrated" and the decision that "the regulatory body should act as if no effect has been demonstrated" (Krewski et al. 1989, p. 9; cf. Leisenring and Ryan 1992). For that purpose tests of significance are completely inappropriate.[3]

The other technical concept referred to above is the *no-observed-effect level* (NOEL), also called the *no-effect level* (NEL), *no-adverse-effect level* (NAEL), or *no-observed-adverse-effect level* (NOAEL). This is the highest experimental dose level that produces no observable adverse effect in the most sensitive animal species. The NOEL of a substance is commonly taken as an indicator of its toxicity. In food toxicology, the NOEL is divided by a "safety factor" (uncertainty factor), typically 100, to arrive at a supposedly tolerable level for humans.

Like the significance concept, the concept of a NOEL is constructed in a way that leads to the neglect of type II errors. If a substance has been studied only in very insensitive experiments (e.g., with small animal groups), then the NOEL will be much higher than if it has been studied in more sensitive experiments. As a result, the more uncertain our knowledge is about a substance, the less protection we can expect from a NOEL-based dose level. An illustrative example of this effect was provided by Crump (1984, p. 856): Suppose that in an experiment with 100 rats per dose, the mean liver fat per animal is 15.1 g in the control group and 18.4 g in the treatment group, with a standard deviation of 10.0 g in each group. Under the assumption of a normal distribution, this difference is statistically significant (even at the more stringent 0.01 level). However, if the same numbers are obtained in a study involving only 25 rats per group, the result will not be statistically significant (even at the 0.10 level). Hence, the tested dose would be called a NOEL according to the smaller but not the larger study.[4]

More generally speaking, the use of NOELs safeguards against type I (false-positive) errors, since the underlying experiments are evaluated that way, but it does not protect against type II (false-negative) errors (Brown and Erdreich 1989). Hence, just like the concept of significance, the NOEL concept has a bias that is in many cases the exact opposite of what the public expects from administrators.

EPISTEMIC ASYMMETRY

Many toxic effects are stochastic rather than deterministic phenomena. Many but not all smokers contract cancer, cardiovascular disease, or obstructive lung disease. Even among persons who have smoked the same number of cigarettes for an equally long period of time, some contract one of these diseases, others not. In this and many other cases, the toxicity of a substance is manifested in an increased frequency of a disease.

This is why *group size* is a key factor in both epidemiology and experimental toxicology. If exposure to a substance increases the frequency of a disease from 0% to 3% of the population, then if we study ten exposed individuals, we cannot be at all sure of seeing a case of the disease. (To be more precise, the probability that we will see it is only 0.26.) If the increase is instead from 20% to 23%, then it is impossible to discover the effect in groups as small as this one.

The chances of detecting harmful effects increase when larger groups are used but, unfortunately, not as much as one might wish. Quite large disease frequencies may go undetected in all studies of feasible size. As a rule of thumb, epidemiological studies can only detect reliably excess relative risks that are about 10% or greater. For the more common types of cancer, such as leukemia and lung cancer, lifetime risks are between 1% and 10%. Therefore, even in the most sensitive studies, lifetime risks smaller than 0.1% or 1% cannot be observed (Vainio and Tomatis 1985).

The same statistical problems affect animal experiments. To detect an increase in the mutation rate of 0.5%, about 8,000,000,000 mice are required. (Weinberg 1972, p. 210).[5] Hence, for purely statistical reasons if nothing else, neither epidemiological studies nor laboratory experiments can provide safe negative conclusions. We therefore have an unfortunate epistemic asymmetry in toxicology: It can often be proved beyond a reasonable doubt that a substance has a particular adverse effect. On the other hand, it can seldom be proved beyond a reasonable doubt that a substance does not have a particular adverse effect, and in practice it can never be proved that it has no adverse effect at all. From the viewpoint of the philosopher of science, this asymmetry of toxicological knowledge gives rise to an interesting problem in falsificationism. According to that doctrine, scientific theories and hypotheses can be empirically falsified but not verified. However, when a toxicologist considers a hypothesis such as "nitromethane is carcinogenic," the opposite situation obtains. This hypothesis can be verified (e.g., by convincing epidemiological studies), but it can never be falsified, since no experiment can exclude a very weak carcinogenic effect. As far as I can see, falsificationism can be saved only at the price of disidentifying the "hypothesis" referred to by the philosopher of science and the hypothesis that a working scientist sets out to test.

This epistemic asymmetry also has important practical consequences. Since no substance can be shown to be non-hazardous, a complete reversal of the conventional scientific burden of proof is impossible (Hansson 1997a). This is an unwelcome conclusion, since it means in practice that no absolute safety can be obtained.

EXPOSURE LIMITS

The preceding discussion implies that there is no reliable scientific basis for drawing a line between hazardous and nonhazardous concentrations of a toxic substance (as opposed, of course, to drawing a line between concentrations with and without *known* hazards). In view of this, it is perhaps surprising that anybody has been willing to provide exposure limits for hazardous chemicals. However, in the early days of occupational standard setting, the epistemological problems outlined above were largely unknown. The knowledge that toxicity is often stochastic, and that important health effects may be impossible to discover, belongs to the modern "epidemiological" era of the science of health.

TABLE 1–1. Overall Levels of 11 National Lists of OELs in Force in 1995

COUNTRY	LEVEL OF OEL LIST IN 1995
Philippines	0.59
Turkey	0.59
United Kingdom	0.32
Australia	0.31
Germany	0.31
Japan	0.29
Finland	0.28
France	0.26
Denmark	0.21
Sweden	0.15
Russia	0.13

The original threshold limit values (TLVs) from 1946 are used as a basis of comparison, so that the Philippine values are on average 59% of the 1946 TLVs (geometric mean). See the Appendix for technical details.

Occupational standard setting was initiated in the "preepidemiological" era.

The first occupational exposure limits were proposed by individual researchers in the 1880s. In the 1920s and 1930s, several lists were published in both Europe and the United States, and in 1930 the Ministry of Labor of the USSR issued what was probably the first official list (Cook 1987, pp. 9–10). In 1946 the American Conference of Governmental Industrial Hygienists (ACGIH) published the first edition of their list. This list, which is revised yearly, has a dominant role as a standard reference for official lists all over the world. Since the 1970s most industrialized countries have developed their own lists of occupational exposure limits.

Table 1.1 and Figure 1.1 compare the average levels of OEL lists in 11 countries in 1995. The ACGIH list from 1946 is used as a basis for

14   SETTING THE LIMIT

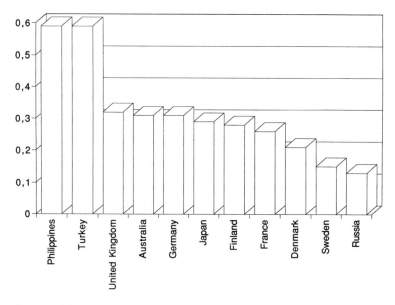

FIGURE 1.1. The overall level of 11 official lists of OELs from 1995. The 1946 list of TLVs has been used as a unit of comparison. See Table 1.1 and the Appendix for details.

comparison. Hence, the Philippine list has the value 0.59. This means that the exposure limits on this list are on average 59% of the corresponding limits on the ACGIH list from 1946. (Comparisons are by geometric means; for technical details, see the Appendix.) Measured in the same way, the 1995 list of the ACGIH would be assigned the value 0.23.

There are large differences between the national lists. The OELs of the Philippines and Turkey are on average about twice as high as those of most Western countries, whereas Denmark and, in particular, Sweden and Russia have lower OELs than most other countries. For a detailed study, I have selected three lists of OELs. One is the list issued by the ACGIH, chosen because of its worldwide influence. The others are the official national lists of Germany and Sweden. For both of these lists, extensive scientific documentation has been published. The

German list is officially declared to be based only on considerations of health, whereas the Swedish list is presented as the outcome of a compromise between health and economic or technological feasibility. The Swedish list seems to have on average the lowest values in the Western world. (The Russian values are of less interest due to a history of "showpiece" exposure limits in the Soviet Union that were seldom complied with.) For our first case study, let us now take a closer look at the threshold limit values.

2

THE MOST INFLUENTIAL VALUES

By far the most influential OELs are the threshold limit values (TLVs) that have been issued yearly since 1946 by the ACGIH. In this chapter, we trace the ideas behind the TLVs and evaluate the achievements and shortcomings of the TLV committee.

THE ACGIH AND ITS TLVs

The ACGIH was founded in 1938 (Paull 1984).[1] In spite of its name, it is a voluntary organization, with no formal ties to government or state authorities in the United States or elsewhere. Originally, its members were federal, state, and local officials in the area of industrial health, but within a few years of its inception, academics and industry consultants were accepted as members (Castleman and Ziem 1988, p. 532). In 1941, it set up a Threshold Limits Subcommittee, and a list of exposure limits, covering about 140 chemical substances, proposed by this committee was adopted by the ACGIH in 1946. Since then the list has been extended and revised, with a new edition published yearly (Paull 1984).

About ten years after its first list was published, the committee started to work on written documentation for the TLVs. In 1962, the first "Documentation of TLVs" was published. For each substance on the list, it contained, a brief summary of its effects, with references and with reasons for choosing the TLV. Revised versions of the documentation volume were published in 1966, 1971, 1980, 1986, and 1991. Since 1980, new and revised documentations for individual substances have been published continuously (Cook 1985, 1987; ACGIH 1990).

In the 1940s and 1950s, the ACGIH and the American Standards Association (ASA) competed for the position of leading setter of occupational health standards. The values of the two organizations did not differ much in numerical terms, but the ASA values were ceiling values below which all workplace concentrations should fluctuate, whereas the ACGIH values were (and still are, with few exceptions) upper limits for the average during a whole work day. Therefore, the ASA standards provided greater protection to exposed workers. The ACGIH won the struggle and emerged in the early 1960s as virtually the only source of exposure limits that practitioners looked to for guidance (Magnuson 1965, p. 544; Sentes 1992, p. 761). How the struggle was won remains to be clarified, but one factor may have been that the ACGIH's values were less demanding and thus easier to implement. Federal and state control of work environments was very weak at the time. Hence, standards were chosen primarily by occupational hygienists hired by industry, whose precarious positions would have been worsened by attempts to implement stricter and more expensive standards.

In 1969, as part of its greater involvement in occupational health, the federal government adopted the 1968 TLVs as an official standard. In the years that followed, the legal process for updating these values or adopting new ones turned out to be extremely slow and resource-consuming. The Occupational Safety and Health Administration (OSHA) was unable to follow the reductions in TLVs undertaken by the ACGIH, let alone make its own reassessments of the values originally adopted. By 1987, OSHA had succeeded in promulgating new regulations for only 26 substances. As a result of this backlog, 234 substances had a lower limit on the list of TLVs than on the official list, and 168 additional substances had TLVs but were not included in the official list (Paull 1984, p. 235; Robinson et al. 1991, p. 4). To catch up, the 1987–88 TLV list was adopted in 1989 as a new official standard.

This decision was heavily attacked from two sides. From one side, OSHA was criticized for not adopting lower and more protective values than the TLVs. The most prominent critic was another federal agency, the National Institute for Occupational Safety and Health (NIOSH). To substantiate its criticism, NIOSH presented toxicity data for 98 substances, which they considered to have insufficiently protective TLVs. For 50 of these substances, NIOSH proposed an exposure limit. These limits were on average 6.1 times lower than the TLVs adopted by OSHA (geometric mean).[2]

From the other side, OSHA was criticized for being too hard on industry. These critics won a legal victory in 1992, when a federal court of appeals overturned OSHA's 1989 decision, requiring the agency to enforce for most substances TLVs from the 1968 list. In 1996, OSHA launched a new procedure designed to revise a limited number of conspicuously outdated exposure limits (Paustenbach 1997).

Throughout the Western world, the TLVs have been the starting point for national standard setting on occupational chemical exposure. They are influential in Argentina, Australia, Austria, Belgium, Brazil, Canada, Chile, Denmark, Germany, India, Indonesia, Ireland, Israel, Japan, Malaysia, Mexico, the Netherlands, the Philippines, Portugal, South Africa, Spain, Sweden, Switzerland, Thailand, the United Kingdom, Venezuela, the former Yugoslavia, and probably many other countries as well.[3]

Despite admonitions to the contrary by the ACGIH, the TLVs are also widely used in the evaluation of possible occupational origins of disease. Referring to American experiences, William Morton reported: "Frequently, one may encounter patients with work-related conditions whose workers' compensation claims are denied, at least partially, on the legal argument that workplace substance measurements have shown only values less than the officially recommended TLVs'' (1988, p. 722; cf. Cullen 1991). In addition, TLVs (divided by safety factors) have been used as the basis for air pollution standards in the United States and elsewhere (Robinson and Paxman 1992).

In 1965, Harold Magnuson explained the success of the TLVs as "due, in part, to their [the ACGIH's] comprehensive listing of all important chemicals and to their willingness to make decisions in the face of incomplete evidence" (p. 544). More recently, Liora Salter has added another explanation: The ACGIH, as a voluntary body, has achieved its position due to a regulatory vacuum (1988, pp. 39–41). If OSHA, after first adopting the TLVs in 1969, had managed to revise and update its list on a regular basis, then the present position of the ACGIH would probably be much weaker.[4] Corporate lawsuits against OSHA and other regulatory agencies have helped to prevent this from happening. Furthermore, the comparative ease with which the TLVs can be implemented has probably contributed to their success. Competing exposure limits such as those of NIOSH are generally more costly and thus give rise to much more opposition from industry.

HEALTH-BASED, REALISTIC OR BOTH?

In 1948, the ACGIH provided the following explanation of what TLVs are intended to achieve:

> People vary greatly in response to drugs and toxic substances. Therefore, it is a figment of the imagination to think that we can set down a precise limit below which there is complete safety and immediately above which there may be a high percentage of cases of poisoning among those exposed. With these facts in mind the Committee has set values below which it is fair to expect reasonable protection and above which it is reasonable to expect that we can have occasional cases of poisoning. (Quoted in Breysse 1991, p. 424)

The 1953 list of TLVs contained a preface stating that TLVs were "maximum average concentrations of contaminants to which workers may be exposed for an 8-hour working day (day after day) without injury to health." In 1958, this formulation was tempered, and TLVs were now said to "represent conditions under which it is believed that nearly all workers may be repeatedly exposed, day after day, without adverse effect" (quoted in Ziem and Castleman 1989, p. 911). This statement has been retained. The preamble of the latest TLV list begins with the following two paragraphs:

> Threshold Limit Values (TLVs) refer to airborne concentrations of substances and represent conditions under which it is believed that nearly all workers may be repeatedly exposed day after day without adverse health effects. Because of wide variation in individual susceptibility, however, a small percentage of workers may experience discomfort from some substances at concentrations at or below the threshold limit; a smaller percentage may be affected more seriously by aggravation of a pre-existing condition or by development of an occupational illness. Smoking of tobacco is harmful for several reasons. Smoking may act to enhance the biological effects of chemicals encountered in the workplace and may reduce the body's defense mechanisms against toxic substances.
>
> Individuals may also be hypersusceptible or otherwise unusually responsive to some industrial chemicals because of genetic factors, age, personal habits (smoking, alcohol, or other drugs), medication, or previous exposures. Such workers may not be adequately protected from adverse health effects from certain chemicals at concentrations at or below the threshold limits. An occupational physician should evaluate the extent to which such workers require additional protection. (ACGIH 1996, p. 3)

The official stance of the TLV committee is, not surprisingly, that the TLVs provide sufficient protection of workers' health. Herbert Stokinger, who was a member of the TLV committee for 26 years and its chairman for 15 years, said in 1988:

> [T]hroughout all the more than 40 years of existence of threshold limit values, there has been no instance of serious health effects, provided exposures were kept at or below the TLVs. This I have been careful to

observe in my more than quarter of a century as TLV Committeeman and Chairman.[5]

On the other hand, the TLV committee has attested to at least two exceptions to its claim that TLVs protect workers' health. First, irritation effects are not covered if tolerance develops with continued exposure. In 1969 Stokinger explicitly warned against basing exposure limits on irritation effects shown on volunteers in exposure chambers:

> Human volunteer exposures. . . . should be repeated, however, with sufficient frequency to determine whether tolerance of sensitivity [*sic*] is a feature of the exposure. It has been the experience of the committee that TLVs of irritants et alia, based on *single* human exposures, all too commonly result in far too severe limits. (p. 278)

Needless to say, the emergence of (subjective) tolerance to irritation effects means that a biological warning signal has been silenced. It does not necessarily follow that the exposure is harmless. One counterexample is "tolerance" of high concentrations of corrosive substances, which can be accompanied by severe lesions in skin and mucous membranes and by acid etching of teeth (Leung and Paustenbach 1988).

The other, probably more important, admitted exception is that TLVs are intended to protect *normal* workers, not those who are more sensitive to toxic substances. This was indicated in the two paragraphs from the preamble quoted above. Stokinger has made it clear that the TLV for asbestos "relates to asbestos alone, and does not embrace the major effects from smoking which cannot be factored out exactly" (1988, p. 231). In other words, asbestos workers who smoke are not protected against the dramatically increased risk of pulmonary cancer, in addition to the risk resulting from smoking alone, arising from this unusually deadly combination of exposures. A former chairman of the ACGIH, Ernest Mastromatteo, has made the following statement:

> As noted earlier, TLVs represent exposure concentrations under which it is believed that nearly all workers will not suffer an adverse health effect with prolonged exposure. TLVs are not designed nor intended to protect

all workers. Some workers are known to be more susceptible than others to the effects of exposure to chemicals for a variety of reasons, including inherited genetic disorders, nutritional deficiencies, parasitic diseases, pre-existing diseases such as bronchial asthma or chronic bronchitis, alcohol and drug consumption, and cigarette smoking. (1981, p. 768)

With this extensive list of exceptions (and we saw a similar list in the preamble quoted above), it is not clear that "normal," and thus protected, workers will in all cases be a majority.[6]

That the TLVs do not protect all workers was underlined by the ACGIH's chairman, Jeffrey S. Lee, in a "message from the chair" in 1987:

> The Committee idealistically functions as occupational health professionals by recommending TLVs to protect the health of workers *without regard to* economic or technical feasibility.
> TLVs unquestionably do not protect all workers. This is clearly stated in the preface of the TLV book, and it is believed, is widely understood by practicing professionals. (p. F7)

It is not easy to reconcile the first and second sentences of this statement. If the TLVs are intended to protect workers, with no regard to economic and technological feasibility, what then can be the rationale for deliberately choosing values that do not protect all workers? Lee provides no clue to an answer.

On the other hand, representatives of the ACGIH have also attributed to the TLVs the virtue of economic and technological realism. Stokinger has criticized the NIOSH values for being "unrealistically low in many cases for industry to conform with" (1984 [1981], p. 277). In the same paper, he warned against "attempts to convert a TLV designed for an eight-hour day into one for thirty minutes, and thus, provide a dangerously excessive limit" (p. 280). On another occasion he wrote:

> Another vexing committee problem arises from the misinterpretation and misuse of TLVs. Particularly culpable are the factory inspector and the legal profession. Their common fault lies in misinterpreting the TLVs as

fine lines between safe and dangerous concentrations "either it is or it isn't" phenomenon. Such strict interpretation is not within the intent expressed in the preface of the TLVs, and places industry in undue jeopardy. ... The reason this is so is that the TLV has an inherent safety zone between the limiting value and the concentration capable of producing injury. (Stokinger 1969, p. 280; see also Stokinger 1984 [1956], p. 89)

If the TLVs were as safe as Stokinger said, then it would not often be necessary to reduce them. However, drastic reductions in the TLVs have taken place over the half century of their existence. As Richard Wedeen aptly remarked, "[t]he only certainty is that the 'safe' level changes with time. Exposure standards have fallen continuously as occupational disease has gained recognition and epidemiological investigations have confirmed the presence of preventable disease" (1991, p. 684). The most dramatic change is the TLV for benzene, which has been reduced in five steps from 100 to 0.1 ppm (Rappaport 1993, p. 689).

Table 2.1 and Figure 2.1 show the average development of the TLVs for the substances included in the first list from 1946. The TLVs of these substances are now on average (geometric mean) less than one-fourth of the original TLVs.[7] It is difficult to reconcile this empirical evidence with the picture often given of the TLVs as representing reliable, safe values.

HARMFUL EFFECTS BELOW THE TLVs

Examples of harmful effects at levels below the TLVs are easily found. Numerous such examples are referred to in the ACGIH's own documentation volumes (Roach and Rappaport 1990). Still more examples can be found in the scientific literature on occupational health. Their frequency was brought out in a rather dramatic way by Grace Ziem and Barry Castleman, who reviewed the contents of four major peer-reviewed journals in occupational medicine for 33 months, from January 1987 to September 1989, and found 31 articles that described

TABLE 2–1. Development of the Overall Level of the TLV List of the ACGIH.

YEAR	LEVEL OF TLVS
1946	1.00
1951	0.74
1956	0.71
1961	0.66
1966	0.59
1971	0.52
1976	0.45
1981	0.35
1986	0.31
1991	0.29
1996	0.23

The level of TLVs has been measured as geometric means of the quotients between the updated values and the values on the original list from 1946. See the Appendix for details.

harmful effects at or below the TLVs. One article reported asthma at half of the TLV for toluene diisocyanate; another, changes in renal function at less than a tenth of the TLV for cadmium; and a third, bone marrow changes and leukemia at a tenth of the TLV for benzene (Ziem and Castleman 1989, pp. 914–915).[8]

Each such example (numerous others can be found in the scientific literature) disproves the 1988 statement by a former ACGIH chairman, quoted above, that no worker has been injured by exposure to chemicals at or below the TLV. Presumably, that statement was based on the information that had reached the TLV committee from its usual sources, rather than on a search of the scientific literature.

Vernon Carter, another former chairman of the ACGIH, has commented on effects below the TLVs as follows:

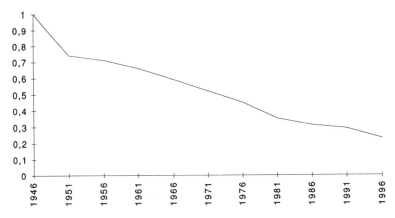

FIGURE 2.1. Development of the ACGIH's TLVs. For details, see Table 2.1 and the Appendix.

The committee is asked many times why a certain TLV seems to ignore a report from field experience which would indicate an adverse response to an exposure level below the established TLV. Although the committee is not perfect and could certainly overlook some published information, that is not usually the case. Much of the field exposure data, especially that found in some of the older literature[,] is very subjective and did not take into account the many variables which could induce the observed response. In addition, the measurement technology used, although the best available at that time, may have been demonstrated to be inaccurate. In our rush to use human data whenever available, we must be careful to apply the same strenuous review of this data that we apply to data from controlled human exposures and animal studies. (Carter 1985, p. 13)

This argument does not hold water (and no other one seems to be available from official ACGIH quarters). Evidence of harmful effects below the TLVs is not found primarily in outdated sources. Instead it is found in scientific articles in the modern peer-reviewed occupational health journals. As Ziem and Castleman have shown, in only four of these journals, such articles seem to be accumulating at the rate of approximately one per month.

THE USE OF CORPORATE INFORMATION

Another study by Castleman and Ziem (1988) indicates that the peer-reviewed scientific literature has a smaller role in the deliberations of the TLV committee than one might expect. The minutes of the committee from 1972 to 1976 showed that the (nonvoting) members who represented chemical manufacturers were responsible for proposing and documenting TLVs for their own companies' products.

Castleman and Ziem also show that according to the ACGIH's documentation volumes from 1986, the TLVs for more than 100 substances relied to a large extent on unpublished corporate information. In the documentation volumes, such information is recorded in the form of brief statements, typically to the effect that a certain level had been found to be safe or that no evidence of damage to health had been found at that level.

Due to sloppy—or rather nonexistent—filing procedures, most of this unpublished corporate information is now unavailable for scientific scrutiny. Some of it never came in written form but transmitted by telephone. Therefore, nothing is known about the methods used for measuring and assessing the exposures or for assessing the health status of the exposed workers. From a scientific point of view, undocumented statements such as these cannot form the basis of valid conclusions.

These practices of the TLV committee must be seen against the historical background. Prior to the 1970s, federal regulation of occupational health and safety was virtually nonexistent, and state agencies lacked power and resources for surveillance of industry (Castleman and Ziem 1988). Therefore, government officials and independent researchers in the United States had no means of accessing information about occupational exposures and health effects other than to ask industry to supply it voluntarily.

The epistemological stance of the committee was, quite naturally, generally the same as the predominant view in occupational medicine. The distinction between epidemiological studies and unsystematic observations was not yet clear. This is why observations such as "We have no health problems here among workers exposed to

300 ppm'' were taken to be valid evidence of the harmlessness of a substance. Although the TLV committee's reliance on unsystematized practical experience was, in its early years, consistent with mainstream occupational hygiene, the committee was somewhat unusual in deemphasizing the role of medical experts in evaluating the health status of workers. The first TLV committee included no physician, and as late as 1966 the Industrial Medical Association publicly complained that too few of the committee members (only 4 out of 12) had a medical education (Golz et al. 1966; Ziem and Castleman 1989, p. 911). The dominating profession was industrial hygiene. In 1947, the committee chairman, L. T. Fairhall, himself a chemist and an industrial hygienist, expressed great confidence in the ability of his own profession to judge the health status of workers:

> The industrial hygienist is in contact with not one, but a number of plants, using a given toxic substance. He knows, as no one else knows, the actual aerial concentration of contaminant encountered in practice. And he is in contact with the individuals exposed and therefore soon learns whether the concentrations measured are causing any injury or complaint. His judgement and the combined judgement of this entire Conference group is therefore most valuable in helping formulate maximum allowable concentration values. (Quoted in ACGIH 1990, p. 340)

In 1969, Stokinger published a description of the committee's procedures that is worth quoting at length:

> Procedures used by the committee take three forms: (1) The chairman and members of the appropriate subcommittee hold a meeting with industry's physicians and industrial hygienists and review their experience. This procedure is used where the data has not been assembled or published. This procedure has been used for the TLVs for the chromate industry and the nitroglycols. (2) Where the data or reports have been published, these are reviewed by the chairman and the committee and the action taken is that mutually agreed upon by industry and the American Conference of Governmental Industrial Hygienists by letter correspondence. This procedure has been used for beryllium, quartz, uranium, and vanadium pentoxide.

(3) Active cooperative projects with industry and [the] toxicology and pathology section of the occupational health program (OHP) are entered into whereby industry supplies the health records or clinical data for review, or active toxicologic research investigations are made by OHP in conjunction with clinical and environmental data obtained by industry. Such is being done cooperatively with a large producer of isocyanates to determine means of detecting the hypersusceptible worker, a side bonus of which will be the validation of the TLV for the isocyanates. A similar study is being cooperatively made of carbon disulfide. (p. 279)

Stokinger's statement that "the action taken is that mutually agreed upon" with industry does not seem consistent with his indignant response, 19 years later, to accusations of corporate influence. "For all my 26 years on the Committee, would I as Chief Toxicologist, U.S. Public Health Service, permit corporate influence to intrude on the impartial character of the American Conference of Governmental Industrial Hygienists (ACGIH)?" (Stokinger 1988 p. 231).

As the documentation volumes show, unpublished information from companies to the effect that specified levels of chemicals give rise to no problems are still a major source of TLVs.[9] To rely on such information means to uphold neither modern standards of epidemiological research nor modern standards of peer review and scientific publishing.

It must be emphasized that corporate information is an important source for risk assessments of chemical substances. Regulators should demand health-related information from companies, and responsible companies should actively provide it to both regulators and researchers. But just like information from any other source, it must be carefully evaluated. In particular, summary statements that are not corroborated by detailed data should not be treated as conclusive evidence.

UNORTHODOX TOXICOLOGY

More than anyone else, Herbert Stokinger has shaped the thinking of the TLV committee. Some of his views on toxicology appear to have been quite unorthodox. In a 1963 article, criticizing the much lower Soviet exposure limits, he wrote:

> As inhaled concentrations become progressively lower to reach the threshold of response as measured by changes in optical chronaxy or light sensitivity or odor response, they approach trace quantities. Trace quantities of substances, rather than acting adversely as interpreted by the Soviets, tend to act beneficially. The toxicologic literature is replete with instances of substances that, though toxic in high concentrations, in trace amounts prove stimulating to growth, reproduction and longevity. Fluoride, iodine and sex hormones are commonly recognized examples; vanadium, uranium, hydrogen sulfide, and even ionizing radiation, are in this category. (p. 472)

The view that "[t]race quantities of substances"—not certain specified substances, but chemical substances in general—tend to act beneficially is unsupported by modern toxicology, and it was equally unsupported when this statement was written. (It prevails, however, in the pseudoscientific doctrine of homeopathy.) True, most if not all substances with beneficial effects are poisonous in larger doses, but from this no such conclusion can be drawn. We seem to have here a fallacious conclusion from

> If a substance is beneficial in small doses, then it is harmful in large doses.

to

> If a substance is harmful in large doses, then it is beneficial in small doses.

This is an example of the classic fallacy of affirming the consequent, against which numerous logicians from Aristotle on have warned us.[10]

Another example of Stokinger's unorthodox toxicology can be found in an article published in 1987, in which he attempted to show that chemical carcinogens have thresholds, i.e., nonzero dose levels below which they do not give rise to cancer. One of his more precise statements to this effect is that vinyl chloride has "a threshold somewhere below 50 and above 10 ppm'' (p. 6). Stokinger claimed that there are three types of evidence for such a threshold: (*1*) human evidence, (*2*) animal evidence referring to cancer incidence, and (*3*) animal evidence of a biochemical nature.

1. The human evidence is that ''more than 35 years have passed since workers were exposed to vinyl chloride containing small amounts (5 ppm) of vinylidene chloride, without the appearance of tumors. Vinyl chloride levels during the 1950's, although averaging 160 ppm, rose occasionally to 1000 ppm at some work operations, but later were around 50 ppm or below. This gives epidemiological evidence of a threshold somewhere below 50 and above 10 ppm'' (Stokinger 1987, p. 6). The reference given for this is a 1972 article by C. G. Kramer and T. E. Mutchler of the Dow Chemical Company.

   Kramer's and Mutchler's findings refer to a group of 98 male workers who had been exposed to vinyl chloride ''for periods [of] up to 25 years'' (p. 19), not for ''more than 35 years.'' No tumors had developed in the group. However, no mention is made of the tumor incidence at any higher dose level. Without such information, no indication of the plausibility of a threshold can be obtained. (It should also be noted that from a statistical point of view, 98 exposed persons is too small a group to exclude risks of cancer that are much too large to be ignored. If, for instance, the true incidence of a disease is 0.7% at a certain level of exposure, then the probability is 0.5 that no case of it will be found in a group of this size.)

2. Stokinger referred to two animal studies ''in which a few tumors were still appearing in rats at 50 ppm, but none at 10 ppm, indicating a threshold somewhere between 50 and 10 ppm'' (1987, p. 6). One of these studies is an article by Keplinger et al. (1975), and the other is an article referred to as ''Maltoni.'' No article by Maltoni appears in the list of references, but in another publication, Stokinger (1984) referred to a paper by C. Maltoni and G. Lefemine (1975) to substantiate the same claim.

The article by Keplinger and coworkers reports tests carried out at the Industrial Bio-Test Laboratories in 1978. In 1983, three officials of this laboratory were convicted of mail fraud. Their crime was to have faked toxicity data on drugs under review by the Food and Drug Administration and the Environmental Protection Agency. One of the three convicted officials was Moreno Keplinger (Marshall 1983). In his 1987 article, Stokinger does not mention the problematic status of experiments reported by Keplinger from this laboratory.

At any rate, Keplinger's article does not contain the information ascribed to it. It describes a study in which rats, mice, and hamsters were exposed to 0, 50, 200, and 2500 ppm vinyl chloride. No animals were exposed to 10 ppm. Angiosarcomas had been discovered at 50 ppm, as Stokinger says, but, of course, no information about effects at 10 ppm can be gained from this study.

The report by Maltoni and Lefemine summarizes a long series of experiments conducted by the authors at the Istituto di Oncologia and the Centro Tumori in Bologna, Italy. A carcinogenic effect had been shown at 50 ppm. No results from exposures below this level were reported. However, a study with exposures to 25, 10, and 5 ppm was described as "just started" (Maltoni and Lefemine 1975, p. 199). In 1981, a final report from this study was published. Among the findings were five liver angiosarcomas among 120 animals at 25 ppm and one liver angiosarcoma among 120 animals at 10 ppm (Maltoni et al. 1981, p. 20). Hence, Stokinger was wrong when he claimed in 1987 that this experiment showed that no tumors appear at 10 ppm.

3. Finally, Stokinger quoted an article by P. G. Watanabe and coworkers at the Dow Chemical Company (1976), maintaining that this article provides "indisputable evidence" of "a threshold for vinyl chloride hemangiomas (tumors) of the rat liver somewhere more than 10 ppm and less than 50 ppm." In this experiment, hepatic nonprotein sulfhydryl was used as an indicator of the body's capacity to neutralize vinyl free radicals. "[A] distinct

dose–response relation was found for exposure levels of 2000, 1000, 250, 150, 50, and 10 ppm. Exposure at the four highest levels caused a progressive depression of the hepatic nonprotein sulfhydryl content, whereas no depression was observed at 10 ppm'' (Stokinger 1987, p. 6).

Stokinger's description of the experiment is correct, but it leaves out two important facts: The exposures were short, and the groups were small. The information about the absence of effects at 10 ppm was based on five animals that had been exposed for 7 hours. No statistically significant effect was discovered in this group. Clearly, a biologically significant effect at 10 ppm might have gone undetected in this very small experiment.

In summary, Stokinger's argument gives us no reason to believe that vinyl chloride has a threshold at the level he proposes. Of course, the substance may have a threshold at this or another level. However, a scientifically well-founded argument for a threshold hypothesis cannot be based primarily on the demonstration that no cases of cancer have been detected at certain exposure levels. Instead, it has to be based on a much more sophisticated understanding of toxicological mechanisms.

CONCLUSIONS

The TLVs of the ACGIH are the most influential occupational exposure limits worldwide. They have the important advantages of covering a large number of substances and of being revised and updated every year. With respect to procedures for updating, the TLVs compare most favorably to the exposure limits officially promulgated by the U.S. government.

On the other hand, the TLVs offer only incomplete protection against adverse health effects, as can be seen from the many scientific reports of such effects below the TLVs. Furthermore, the scientific standard of the underlying documentation is not impressive, and many TLVs are still based on information that has not passed and could not pass the peer-review system of modern journals of occupational health.

Our next case is the German commission for occupational exposure limits. Since this is a subcommittee of the German research council, high scientific standards should be expected.

3

PURELY HEALTH-BASED VALUES?

The official German list of OELs is published yearly by the Commission for the Investigation of Health Hazards of Chemical Compounds in the Work Area (Senatskommission zur Prüfung gesundheitsschädlicher Arbeitsstoffe) of the Deutsche Forschungsgemeinschaft (Senatskommission 1996b). The values on this list are called *maximum workplace concentrations* (*Maximale Arbeitsplatzkonzentrationen*, MAK). To substantiate them, extensive documentation reports are published (Senatskommission 1995).

The MAKs are said to be based exclusively on scientific information about health effects and thus to be unaffected by economic, political, or technological considerations. The main purpose of this chapter is to evaluate this claim of scientific purity. The evaluation is based on a reading of the documentation reports that have been issued for the MAKs (about 4200 pages). It is restricted to MAKs and thus does not include the corresponding documentation for standards used in *biological monitoring (Biologische Arbeitsstofftoleranzwerte*, BAT).

IN WHAT SENSE HEALTH-BASED?

To begin with, the term *health-based* needs to be clarified and operationalized. According to the preamble of the MAK list, a MAK is "defined as the maximum concentration of a chemical substance (as gas, vapor or particulate matter) in the workplace air which generally does not have known adverse effects on the health of the employee nor cause unreasonable annoyance even when the person is repeatedly exposed during long periods, given a 40-hour working week (or 42-hour when averaged over four weeks in firms with four work shifts)" (Senatskommission 1996b, p. 9, and 1996a, p. 9) Furthermore:

> MAK values are established on the basis of the effects of chemical substances; when possible, practical aspects of the industrial processes and the resulting exposure patterns are also taken into account; scientific criteria for the prevention of adverse effects on health are decisive, not technical or economical feasibility. (Senatskommission 1996b, p. 9, and 1996a, p. 9)

All new members of the MAK commission receive a letter from the president of the Deutsche Forschungsgemeinschaft that specifies their mission. This letter emphasizes that "extrascientific problems" such as political and economic consequences have no place in the determination of MAKs (Senatskommission 1996b, p. 188, and 1996a, p. 180). Dietrich Henschler, a previous chairman of the commission, asserts that "[s]ocial, economic and technical parameters are expressly excluded" and that the MAKs "represent medical standards, aiming at exclusion of impairment of health, rather than at compromise values at the socioeconomic level" (Henschler 1984, p. 90; cf. Woitowitz 1988, p. 226). Zielhuis and Wibowo (1991) refer to the MAKs as "purely health-based."

Carcinogens and genotoxic substances receive special treatment in the German system. Since 1976, substances in these categories for which MAKs cannot be determined are instead assigned a *technical exposure limit* (*Technische Richtkonzentration*, TRK). In the words of the MAK list:

> TRK values are not MAK values; even observance of TRK cannot fully exclude potential danger to health. (Senatskommission 1996b, p. 123, and 1996a, p. 117)

According to Henschler, this practice was adopted because "the present theory of chemical carcinogenesis indicates that even the lowest doses will produce some genotoxic damage irrespective of the observation or non-observation of tumor formation in finite experimental conditions" (1991, p. 15). Hence, in contrast to the MAKs, the TRKs are not claimed to be based exclusively on considerations of health.

The notion of a purely health-based value can be interpreted in either of the following two ways, which one should distinguish carefully between:

a value that offers complete protection against adverse health effects (*strictly health protective value*)

and

a value that has been based exclusively on information about health effects (*health criteria–based value*).

For practical purposes, strictly health protective values may be seen as a special case of health criteria–based values. A health criteria–based value may, depending on the criteria used to assess health information, provide more or less protection against adverse health effects. In particular, it may (in contrast to a strictly health-protective value) offer less protection than a value based on a compromise between health considerations and economic or technological feasibility (Lundberg et al. 1991).

The use of exposure limits that are not strictly health protective will have to depend on nonhealth objectives that make a compromise necessary. This, of course, applies to health criteria–based values that are not strictly health protective. Such values are the outcome of a compromise, but one that is not established separately for each substance. Instead, the health-based criteria that are applied to all substances have been determined in a way that strikes a balance between health and feasibility. (Whether or not this is better than the alternative method—compromising separately for each substance—will be discussed in Chapter 5.)

A cursory reading of the preamble of the MAK list may give the impression that its values are strictly health protective. A closer reading, especially a study of the documentation reports, will show that this is not the case. Most of the MAK values are (of necessity) based on glaringly incomplete toxicity information. Important potentially harmful effects have not been studied, and even for those that have, reliable negative conclusions are often far beyond the limits of the empirical evidence. Moving from "this effect has not been shown" to "this effect does not exist" generally cannot be done with confidence.

Perhaps the clearest proof that the MAK values are not strictly health protective is the large number of cases in which MAKs had to be reduced to avoid previously unknown adverse health effects. Each such case is proof that the original value was not strictly health protective (although it may, of course, have been so considered). The commission itself presented one such example in its report on 2,4,6-trinitrotoluene (1988):[1]

> The MAK value of 1.5 mg/m^3, which has been valid until now, was adopted from the TLV list in 1958. In 1978 the TLV value was reduced to 0.5 mg/m^3 because of the liver parameter changes observed after 0.8 mg/m^3 exposures. In view of the frequency of dermatitis after exposures between 0.3 and 0.6 mg/m^3 and the reduced erythrocyte numbers at 0.48 mg/m^3, this value also seems to be too high. Cataract formation was observed after prolonged exposure to 0.1–0.35 mg/m^3.... Until biological monitoring data become available, the MAK value will be provisionally reduced to 0.1 mg/m^3.[2]

Even for well-known adverse effects, such as the acute effects of sulfur dioxide on the airways, the dose–effect information on which MAKs were based has turned out to require correction. In its report on sulfur dioxide (1974), the commission wrote:

> The now valid MAK value of 5 ppm = 13 mg/m^3 is intended to protect most workers from the emergence of irritative effects in the airways and to prevent impairments in respiratory function. However, it is possible that this concentration gives rise to a small and completely reversible irritative effect primarily in unaccustomed workers.

The MAK (5 ppm) was retained. Seven years later, in a new report on the same substance (1981), the commission amended its previous conclusion:

> At concentrations of about 5 to 10 ppm most SO$_2$-unaccustomed persons will experience irritative effects in the upper airways and a small to moderate increase in respiratory resistance, and a few sensitive individuals will even have bronchospasms. . . . Slight functional changes can still be shown at exposures to 2.5 and 3 ppm SO$_2$. At 1 ppm SO$_2$ the changes in respiratory resistance and in expiratory flow are at most small, or are not at all present. Due to the expected pathophysiological effects of the described functional changes the MAK value is reduced from 5 ppm to 2 ppm.

Examples such as these show that the MAKs are not strictly health protective.[3] However, they might still be so in the following, greatly weakened sense:

> a value that offers complete protection against all *known* adverse health effects.

We will now investigate whether or not the MAKs satisfy this criterion. After that, we will return to the question of whether they are health criteria–based.

IRRITATION AND WORSE

Many of the documentation reports refer to studies that describe adverse effects at levels below the chosen MAK—for example, to irritation of the eyes and upper airways. However, only in the following few cases were these effects mentioned in the final summary in which the commission explained its choice of an MAK:

Acetaldehyde is a colorless liquid that is used as an intermediate in chemical synthesis.

In a document on acetaldehyde (1971) results from short-term experiments were reported in which 200 ppm gave rise to irritation of the nose and throat in human subjects, and 50 ppm to irritation of the eyes. In spite of this, the MAK value of 200 ppm was not reduced. The information gained from these experiments was said to be insufficient since it was "only concerned with olfactory nuisance and local irritation," and neither "field experiences nor results from long-term exposures" were available. (The MAK was reduced in 1982 due to effects in laboratory animals on respiratory epithelia. MAK 1996: 50 ppm)

Allyl propyl disulfide is a yellow liquid and a major constituent of onion oil. It is used as a food additive.

Writing about this substance (1979), the commission said that the chosen MAK of 2 ppm was related to "the acute irritative effects on mucous membranes." The only dose-related information that was given about this effect referred to a paper (Feiner et al. 1946) according to which workplace concentrations of 1.7–3.4 ppm gave rise to "strong irritation of eyes, nose, and throat." (MAK 1996: 2 ppm)

Acetone is a colorless liquid that has many uses in the chemical industry, including the manufacture of plastics and paints.

In 1993, the MAK for acetone was reduced from 1000 to 500 ppm "due to the clear irritation and nuisance reactions at 1000 ppm, but the slight and reversible reactions, that are not even present in all persons, in the domain of about 500 ppm." (MAK 1996: 500 ppm)

Hence, in 1971 irritation that disappeared after habituation was accepted, and even in 1993 "slight and reversible reactions, that are not even present in all persons" were accepted.[4]

In some reports from the early 1970s, health effects much more serious than irritation were explicitly accepted:

Tetrachloroethylene is a colorless liquid that is used as a solvent and as a degreasing agent for metals.

In 1972, the commission wrote: "The determination of the MAK at 100 ppm is at present not sufficiently well-founded. A couple of minutes at this concentration gives rise to irritation of the mucous membranes. Repeated 7-hour exposures at the same concentration are followed by a series of phenomena that are triggered by effects on the vegetative and central nervous system, and at the same time tetrachloroethylene is accumulated in the organism. Field experiences from prolonged exposures at concentrations around the MAK are not available, and neither are reliable data on the pharmacokinetics of the substance and of its metabolites. Findings from animal experiments indicate that repeated exposure to such concentrations can lead to pathological changes in the liver (e.g. fatty change)." (MAK 1996: 50 ppm)

Carbon disulfide is a liquid that is used as a solvent and as a raw material in various chemical processes, such as the production of textile fibers.

In 1975, the commission wrote: "Long-lasting (5–25 years, on average 11 years) employment in workplace exposures around 20 ppm (now and then between 10 and 40 ppm) leads to a significant increase in systolic and diastolic blood pressure, increased frequency of coronary disease (angina pectoris), and heart-related death; furthermore plasma creatinine is elevated and glucose tolerance is decreased. Several years' work in concentrations between 10 and 20 ppm (partly barely below 10 ppm) leads to impaired psychological performance, hypertension, coronary disease, changes in lung function, and changes in clinical-chemical parameters in blood and urine as well as in neurophysiological measurements. Endocrine or cardiovascular and nervous disturbances can even appear after many years (5–10 resp. 39 years) in concentrations below 10 ppm.... An evaluation of both clinical findings and findings from animal experiments provides reasons to set the MAK at 10 ppm.... This MAK should be seen as provisional." (MAK 1996: 10 ppm)

Thiram is a white powder that is used in the rubber industry and as a fungicide.

The commission wrote in 1976: "Professional contact for 7 days with concentrations much below the MAK value of 5 mg/m^3 gave rise to hypotension and changes in blood count. In animal experiments a week's exposure to concentrations below this value was followed by inflammations in the respiratory tract, aberrations of the menstrual cycle, and disturbances of reproduction. Moderate skin contact was the cause of irritation and inflammation, partly of allergic origin, which was confirmed in animal experiments. Results from other animal experiments are only of limited value for the estimation of risks at the workplace, since in part unrealistic doses were used. For the clarification of the issue of whether the present limit [5 mg/m^3] provides sufficient safety, in particular field experiences of the tolerability of low concentrations are missing, and so are long-term animal studies, primarily inhalation experiments." The MAK value of 5 mg/m^3 was retained. (MAK 1996: 5 mg/m^3)

To the extent that the commission's summaries of the available scientific information are correct, these three MAKs fall far short of protecting human health. Two of these MAKs are still unchanged.

The closest that the commission comes to setting precise standards for the acceptability or nonacceptability of minor adverse effects is its reference in several reports to *work capacity* as a criterion of acceptance.[5] In a report on 1,1,1-trichloroethane (1971) that led up to a MAK of 200 ppm, the commission said:

Decisive for the establishment [of a MAK] are experimental studies in humans, according to which several hours of exposure to 500 ppm gives rise, also when repeated, to slight subnarcotic (sedative) effects that can impair work capacity.

Writing about ethylene glycol dinitrate (1981), the commission said:

> At 0.25 ppm, which has for a long time been accepted as the MAK value, several accounts agree in reporting high incidences of hypotension and headache, and also of subjective indisposition and dizziness. These effects are well known as pharmacological effects of nitro compounds. For the assessment on the workplace *they must be seen as unwanted toxic effects, since they impair work capacity.* (Emphasis added)

To avoid these effects, the MAK was reduced to 0.05 ppm. The quoted passage gives the impression that health effects such as hypotension and headaches are regarded as ''unwanted toxic effects'' only because they reduce the capacity to work. (The surrounding text provides no cue to why the seemingly superfluous attribute ''unwanted'' was added to ''toxic effects.'')

Effect on work capacity was the reason given for two reductions in the MAK for toluene: first from 200 to 100 ppm (1985) and then from 100 to 50 ppm (1993). Arguing for the second of these reductions, the commission said that ''data on effects on work capacity speak for the assumption of first effects (LOAEL) [lowest observed adverse effect level] at about 75 ppm.'' The new value, 50 ppm, was chosen as a level at which ''disturbances of work capacity and of well-being will not appear.''

Hence, as late as in 1993, work capacity seems to have been a factor of some role in the commission's deliberations. The more exact nature of that role cannot be inferred from the documentation reports.

THE PROTECTION OF SUBPOPULATIONS

The definition of MAKs in the opening paragraph of the preamble of the list of MAKs (quoted above) refers to the values as protecting ''the health of the employee.'' Seven pages later, the following restriction is made:

MAK values are established for healthy persons of working age. (Senatskommission 1996b, p. 16, and 1996a, p. 15)

This seems to indicate that no protection of *persons with impaired health* is intended. Nevertheless, at least in one case, the commission has tried to protect such a group. In a report on carbon monoxide (1975), the commission said that 50 ppm would give rise to a carboxyhemoglobin (CO-Hb) level of 5–6%. They acknowledged that adverse health effects were to be expected in persons with angina pectoris at and below that value, but this did not seem to influence their choice of a MAK: "With the now valid MAK value at 50 ppm (55 mg/m^3) healthy workers are protected from impairments of health."

Six years later (1981), a new document was issued on carbon monoxide, saying: "The data now available show that with a carboxyhemoglobin of 2.7% the symptoms of a clinically manifest angina pectoris are intensified; the same applies to patients with peripheral occlusive arterial disease (claudicatio intermittens)." The old value of 50 ppm was still said to "protect healthy persons from impairments of health." To protect persons with angina and claudication, the MAK was reduced to 30 ppm. However, this value was said to correspond to a CO-Hb level of about 4%, which is clearly above the level reported to give rise to the symptoms.

The 1981 reduction in the MAK for carbon monoxide is difficult to understand if we assume that no considerations other than health were taken into account. The reason for the reduction was that the previous value did not protect against certain effects (aggravation of angina and claudication), yet the reduction stopped short of levels at which these effects would have been eliminated. This is easy to understand if the reduction was impeded by economic or technological concerns; otherwise, it is not.

The statement in the preamble, quoted above, says nothing about the protection of *subpopulations who do not have impaired health*, such as those with a deviant metabolism that does not affect their health prior to workplace exposure. A few of the documentation reports discuss this problem directly in regard to the determination of a MAK.

Writing about trichloroethylene (1976), the commission noted that about 10% of humans are unusually sensitive to this substance (due to a difference in the formation and excretion of trichloroethanol). The MAK, they said, should protect this group as well.

The protection of women was at issue in a report on lead (1977). Here the commission referred to a 1976 German law according to which women younger than 45 years of age are not allowed in employment that leads to "an increase of lead in blood to values above 40 µg/100ml." According to the commission, "this restriction applies not only to the protection of the unborn children but also to the women themselves, since their sensitivity to lead is higher than that of men." Detailed biochemical arguments were given for women's higher susceptibility to lead. For workers not covered by the 1976 law (i.e., women at least 45 years old and all men), a MAK value was determined to avoid a lead concentration in blood above 60 µg/100 ml. The commission argued as follows:

> Since there is no sufficiently grounded suspicion that chronic exposure of male employees impairs health at levels below this concentration in blood, the commission does not at present see any reason to consider a lower value.

Hence, women of all ages were said to need stricter protection against lead than men, but the regulations provide that stricter protection only for women below 45 years of age. This discrepancy is not explained in the report; indeed, there is no indication that the commission paid any attention to it.

PROTECTING THE UNBORN

The commission has carefully documented the effects of chemicals on the unborn children of pregnant workers. However, to deal with these risks, they have not chosen the most straight-forward regulatory method—reducing the MAKs whenever necessary to protect the unborn. Instead, separate warnings against embryotoxic effects are printed in the list of MAKs. The preamble explicitly warns that the "observance of [MAK and BAT values] does not guarantee, in every case, that the unborn child is reliably protected from the prenatal toxicity of these substances" (Senatskommission 1996b, p. 16, and 1996a, p. 16). Methyl mercury is assigned a warning ("Group A"): "Exposure of pregnant women can lead to damage to the developing organism even when MAK and BAT values are observed" (Senatskommission 1996b, pp. 16, 74, and 1996a, pp. 16, 69). Sixteen substances are assigned a somewhat weaker warning ("Group B"): "Damage to the developing organism cannot be excluded when pregnant women are exposed, even when MAK and BAT values are observed" (Senatskommission 1996b, pp. 16, 20–100, and 1996a, pp. 16, 20–95).

One of the 16 group B substances is dimethylformamide. In its report on this substance (1992), the commission said that 150 ppm produces embryotoxic effects in rabbits. The no-effect level was reported to be 50 ppm. The MAK value assigned to the substance was 10 ppm, with the following comment:

> The safety margin to the MAK value is too small to make it possible to rule out, in practice, embryotoxic effects even when the MAK value is complied with. Therefore DMF is included in Group B.

Hence, the commission has chosen to warn that certain MAK values do not protect the unborn rather than to reduce these values to protective levels (or to relegate standard setting to technological considerations, as it has done for genotoxic carcinogens). It is difficult to see how this regulatory strategy could be based on health factors alone. On the contrary, it follows naturally from considerations of feasibility. Presumably, removing pregnant women from workplaces with exposures dangerous to the fetus is easier than reducing all workplace exposures to levels at which these dangers are eliminated. Unfortunately, due to the time lag between conception and the recognition of pregnancy, this method does not protect against effects in the sensitive early part of pregnancy. Birth defects due to disturbances of organogenesis occur during the fourth to nineth weeks, when the pregnancy is often unknown (Weeks et al. 1991, pp. 489–501; Peters and Garbis-Berkvens 1996, pp. 935–936).

MARGINS OF SAFETY AND UNSAFETY

We have now tested the hypothesis that the MAKs have been developed to protect against all known adverse health effects. We found that the commission has set several MAKs at levels at which it believes adverse effects occur, and that it does so systematically for embryotoxic effects. Hence, the hypothesis is false: The MAKs have *not* been designed to protect against all known adverse health effects.

Our next task is to test the (weaker) hypothesis that the MAKs are based exclusively on health criteria. To begin with, we need to develop an operative version of that hypothesis. For that purpose, we can use the following consequence of our basic hypothesis:

> HC1 If the information about health effects is the same for two substances, then these substances are treated the same way.

As it stands, HC1 is not yet operative, since there are in practice no two substances for which the information about health effects is exactly the same. However, many MAKs have been established explicitly to protect against a particular effect, which is presumably the adverse effect that appears at the lowest exposure level. Calling this the *critical effect* (Nordberg et al. 1988), we can then modify HC1 as follows:

> HC2 If the commission considers two substances to have the same critical effect, then these substances are treated the same way.

In most cases when two substances have the same critical effect, this effect appears at different concentrations. We will therefore restrict our attention to cases in which the commission mentions not only the critical effect, but also a reference level specifying the concentration at which the effect will appear. For these cases, the following further elaboration of HC2 can be applied:

> HC3 If the commission considers two substances to have the same critical effect, and specifies reference levels for the same degree of this effect, then the ratio between the MAK and the reference level is approximately the same for these two substances.

The quotient between the MAK and the reference level will be called the *regulatory ratio* (RR). Hence, if a MAK of 10 ppm is based on an observation of the presence or absence of a health effect at 100 ppm, then the regulatory ratio is 0.1.[6]

The comparison of regulatory ratios for different substances is complicated by the fact that reference levels may be different in kind. In particular, they may (*1*) refer either to humans or to other species and may (*2*) be either the lowest level at which adverse effects were observed or the highest level at which adverse effects were not observed. We therefore have four types of regulatory ratios, based on reference levels that are

human no-observed-effect levels,

human effect levels,

animal no-observed-effect levels, or

animal effect levels.

Taking this further complication into account, we arrive at the final version of our hypothesis:

> HC4 If the commission considers two substances to have the same critical effect, and specifies reference levels of the same type that refer to the same degree of this effect, then the ratio between the MAK and the reference level is approximately the same for these two substances.

Purely Health-Based Values? 49

HC4 is both an operative and a fairly straightforward consequence of the more basic hypothesis that the MAK values are based exclusively on health criteria. The criteria documents were searched for cases in which a MAK was based explicitly on a critical effect and a reference level in one of these four categories. Cases in the first category turned out to be very difficult to distinguish from more general statements that a MAK represents a safe level of exposure. For the other three categories, a substantial number of cases were found. In what follows, they will be used to test hypothesis HC4.

HUMAN EFFECT LEVELS

In the following eight cases, the MAK was based on adverse effects in humans at specified levels of inhalational exposure. These cases are summarized in Figure 3.1.

Cyclohexane is a constituent of crude oil and of various petroleum products. It is used as a solvent in the paint industry.
   The commission reported (1971) an experiment in rabbits (Treon et al. 1943) in which "[t]he harmless concentration of cyclohexane" was between 435 and 786 ppm. Based on this information, the commission concluded that "[t]he MAK value could therefore probably be set at 400 or 500 ppm." In spite of this, the previous MAK of 300 ppm was retained due to information that "already 300 ppm is somewhat irritative on mucous membranes." RR = 300/300 = 1.0. (MAK 1996: 200 ppm)

2-Hexanone is a colorless liquid that is used primarily as a solvent.
   In 1975, the commission wrote: "In chronic exposure on humans, concentrations from 6 ppm give rise to polyneuritis.... The MAK value is therefore set at 5 ppm for the time being." RR = 0.83. (MAK 1996: 5 ppm)

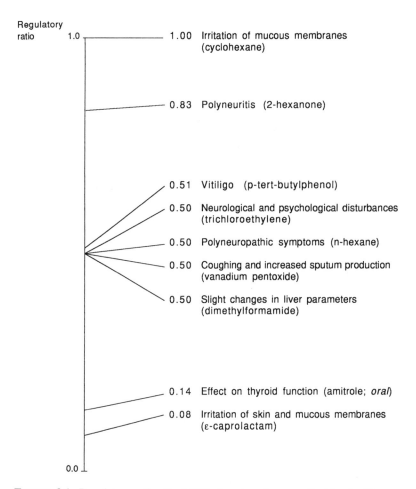

FIGURE 3.1. Regulatory ratios for MAKs based on human effect levels. The effect levels refer to respiratory exposure except in the single case marked "oral."

p-tert-Butylphenol (ptBP) is a crystalline substance that is used in the production of various resins.

The commission settled in 1980 for a "provisional" MAK value of 0.5 mg/m^3 due to a published report (Ebner et al. 1979) showing that "still at values not above 0.96 mg/m^3 ptBP 10 persons with vitiligo were found among 34 exposed workers in a resin factory." RR = 0.5/0.98 = 0.51. (MAK 1996: 0.5 mg/m^3.)

Trichloroethylene is a colorless liquid that is used in metal degreasing and as a solvent.

"Decisive" for a reduction to 50 ppm in 1976 were reports "according to which, at average concentrations of trichloroethylene (over the working week) of 100 ppm disturbances of the central nervous system were observed in the form of a so-called 'psycho-organic syndrome' with neurological impairments and psychological changes as well as visual disturbances." RR = 50/100 = 0.5. (The MAK was 50 ppm until 1996, when it was removed from the list due to a new classification of the substance as a carcinogen.)

n-Hexane is a colorless liquid and an ingredient of many petroleum-based solvents.

In 1982, the MAK was reduced to 50 ppm since "the human organism can react with polyneuropathic symptoms at as little as 100 ppm." RR = 50/100 = 0.5. (MAK 1996 = 50 ppm)

Vanadium pentoxide (V_2O_5) is a yellow to brown crystalline substance. It is used as a catalyst in chemical synthesis and as a photographic developer. Exposure to this chemical also occurs during the cleaning of oil-fired burners due to the presence of vanadium in fuel oils.

A study by Zenz and Berg (1967) was decisive for the adoption in 1985 of 0.05 mg/m^3 as the MAK. "In their study, a single 8 hour exposure of volunteers to as little as 0.1 mg/m^3 V_2O_5 dust resulted in coughing and increased sputum production." RR = 0.05/0.1 = 0.5. (MAK 1996: 0.05 mg/m^3)

Dimethylformamide is a colorless liquid that is used as a solvent and as a raw material in the production of synthetic fibers.

In 1992, the MAK was set at 10 ppm since "indications can be found in the available epidemiological studies that under workplace conditions with 20 ppm small changes can occur in liver parameters." RR = 10/20 = 0.5. (MAK 1996 = 10 ppm)

ε-Caprolactam is a white solid that is used primarily in the production of synthetic fibers.
In 1990, the commission wrote: "The MAK value of ε-caprolactam is determined by the irritation of skin and mucosa caused by the substance in man. It is relatively well documented for ε-caprolactam vapour: 66 mg/m³ has irritant effects, 56 mg/m³ is the irritation threshold and 33 mg/m³ is not irritating. ε-Caprolactam dust has irritant effects on the skin at 84 mg/m³ and on mucous membranes at 61 mg/m³. The effects of lower concentrations have not been described in the literature. To avoid local irritation, therefore, the MAK value of 25 mg/m³ for ε-caprolactam dust and vapour is lowered to 5 mg/m³." RR = 5/61 = 0.08. (MAK 1996: 5 mg/m³)

In one case (also included in Figure 3.1), a regulatory ratio can be calculated from information about effects of oral exposure in humans that was decisive for the MAK.

Amitrole is a water-soluble crystalline solid that is used as an herbicide.
In 1983, the commission wrote: "On the assumption that inhaled amitrole is totally absorbed by the respiratory system, a MAK value of 0.2 mg/m³ air is equivalent to a daily dose for the worker of about 2 mg (equivalent to about 0.03 mg/kg body weight). This dose is less than the threshold dose for an effect on thyroid function and includes a sufficient safety margin (a factor of about 7)." RR = 1/7 = 0.14. (MAK 1996: 0.2 mg/m³)[7]

As Figure 3.1 shows, in seven of the nine cases the regulatory ratio was 0.5 or higher. This corresponds to ''safety factors'' of 2 or less. When ''safety factors'' as small as these are applied to levels that are known to have adverse effects in humans, the resulting MAKs cannot be expected to eliminate these effects in all cases.

One would expect the regulatory ratio to be inversely related to the severity of the critical effect. However, no such correlation can be found in Figure 3.1. The "standard" ratio of 0.5 was connected with health effects as diverse as coughing and increased sputum production (vanadium pentoxide), and psychoneurological disturbances (trichloroethylene). The ratio was as high as 0.83 for polyneuritis associated with 2-hexanone and as low as 0.08 for the irritative effects of ε-caprolactam.[8]

ANIMAL NO-EFFECT LEVELS

When a NOEL is known from inhalation experiments in animals, the conventional approach in standard setting is to perform an interspecies extrapolation of the NOEL from animals to humans.[9] In the following 13 cases, such an extrapolation was the explicit basis for the choice of an MAK. These cases are summarized in Figure 3.2. (On the reliability of some of these NOELs, see the section on "Standards of Evidence.")

Trichlorofluoromethane is a gas (a Freon). Its major uses are as a refrigerant, a solvent, and an aerosol propellant.

The commission wrote in 1989: "In rabbits the 'no effect level' with respect to embryotoxic effects is 1000 ppm for inhalation. . . . The previous MAK value of 1000 ppm will be retained." RR = 1000/1000 = 1.0. (MAK 1996: 1000 ppm)

Butoxydiglycol is a colorless liquid that is used as a solvent and as a constituent of glues and paints.

In their document on this substance (1992), the commission reported: "In studies of inhalation toxicity [in rats], air concentrations of 100 mg/m^3 for 6 hours per day was a no-effect exposure. This was the vapour saturation concentration, i.e. vapours of butoxydiglycol have no deleterious effect. Local damages resulted after

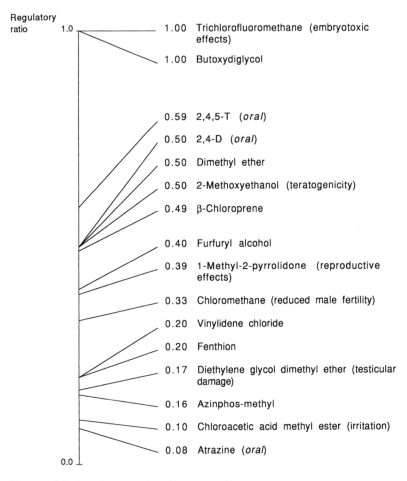

FIGURE 3.2. Regulatory ratios for MAKs based on animal NOELs. The NOELs refer to respiratory exposure except in the three cases marked "oral." The critical effect (against which the NOEL is intended to protect) is indicated when it is clearly identified in the documentation report.

exposure to concentrations above vapour saturation, that is, after inhalation of aerosols (350 mg/m^3). The local deposition of the material is then pathogenic. In practice, exposures to butoxydiglycol at the experimental concentrations of 350 and 1000 mg/m^3 are not to be expected. The MAK value for butoxydiglycol is therefore set at 100 mg/m^3." RR = 100/100 = 1.00. (MAK 1996: 100 mg/m^3)

Dimethyl ether is a gas that is used in plastics production and as a propellant for aerosols.

According to the commission's report (1988), the MAK value was based on animal experiments in which "2000 ppm had no effects. The MAK value can therefore be set at 1000 ppm...." RR = 1000/2000 = 0.50. (MAK 1996: 1000 ppm)

2-Methoxyethanol is a colorless liquid that has multiple uses as an industrial solvent.

According to the commission (1982), rabbits "proved to be the most sensitive of the laboratory animals which have been used, the no adverse effect level for testis damage being about 30 ppm and for teratogenicity between 10 und 50 ppm." The MAK was set at 5 ppm. RR = 5/10 = 0.50. (MAK 1996: 5 ppm)

β-*Chloroprene* is a colorless liquid that is used in the rubber industry.

In 1994, the commission wrote: "For reasons of protection the MAK is reduced to 18 mg/m^3, due to the no-effect concentration in hamster that has been determined to be 37 mg/m^3." RR = 18/37 = 0.49. (MAK 1996: 18 mg/m^3)

Furfuryl alcohol is a liquid that is colorless but turns red or brown when exposed to light. It is used in the production of resins.

The commission reported in 1992: "Since the LC50 [concentration that kills half of the animals] is 85 ppm in rats that are the most sensitive of the studied species, the 'no effect level' for the acute toxicity of furfuryl alcohol must be clearly below this value. Only negligible effects were found in rats subjected to subacute exposure at 19 ppm, under conditions comparable to those at a workplace. In subchronic experiments, neurotoxic effects were no longer found in rats at 25 ppm (NOEL). Since no studies are available of the sensitivity of man to furfuryl alcohol in relation to rats, the MAK value must for safety reasons be set below this concentration. It will be set at 10 ppm and is in need of further substantiation."

Based on the NOEL of 25 ppm, the RR is 10/25 = 0.40. However, since effects were reported at 19 ppm ("uneasiness at the beginning of the experiment and sleepiness throughout the duration of the exposure"), this choice of a NOEL is controversial. It is also noteworthy that an exposure less than nine times higher than the MAK killed half of the exposed rats. (MAK 1996: 10 ppm)

1-Methyl-2-pyrrolidone (NMP) is a liquid that is used as a solvent in the chemical industry and as a cleaner in the production of microelectronic components.

In a 1993 report, the commission concluded that the reproductive effects were decisive for the MAK. "At 206 mg/m^3 (50 ppm) no effects were observed. Therefore, the MAK value for NMP vapours is set at 80 mg/m^3 (20 ppm)." RR = 80/206 = 0.39. (MAK 1996: 80 mg/m^3)

Chloromethane is a gas that has many uses in the chemical industry.

The commission concluded in 1992 that the "no-effect level" for reduction of male fertility was 150 ppm. The MAK was retained at 50 ppm. RR = 50/150 = 0.33. (MAK 1996: 50 ppm)

Vinylidene chloride (VDC) is a colorless liquid that is used primarily in the production of plastics.

In its first report on this substance (1979), the commission said: "In mice, chronic toxic hepatic and renal damage was described after inhalation of 25 ppm VDC. At this dose, which was associated with chronic-toxic changes in organs, VDC gives rise to renal adenocarcinomas, primarily in male mice." The MAK was set at 10 ppm.

In a second report on the same substance (1985), the commission again referred to the same results at 25 ppm and added that 10 ppm did not cause renal or hepatic damage or renal adenocarcinomas in these animals. The tumors observed at 25 ppm were said to be "most probably specific for the strain and sex. . . . The tumors may very well, rather than being genotoxic, be caused by non-specific mechanisms that result from severe toxic damage to the kidneys, and are accompanied by compensatory growth." However: "Due to the small distance between non-toxic as well as toxic and carcinogenic action in Swiss mice the MAK value of 10 ppm is . . . lowered to 2 ppm." (See the section on "Standards of Evidence" for a discussion of the reliability of this NOEL value.) RR = 2/10 = 0.20. (MAK 1996: 2 ppm)

Fenthion is a yellow liquid and an insecticide.
In 1981, the commission wrote: "In subchronic inhalation experiments in rats 1.0 mg/m^3 was without effect." The chosen MAK was 0.2 mg/m^3. RR = 0.2/1.0 = 0.20. (MAK 1996: 0.2 mg/m^3)

Diethylene glycol dimethyl ether is a solvent that is used in the semiconductor industry.
According to the commission's report (1994), the NOEL on rats for damage to testes was 30 ppm, and the MAK was set at 5 ppm. RR = 5/30 = 0.17. (MAK 1996: 5 ppm)

Azinphos-methyl is a brown waxy solid that is used as an insecticide.
In 1976, the commission wrote: "In rats, with repeated exposure to aerosols, the highest concentration with no effect was 1.24 mg/m^3. Therefore, and based on analogies with other organic pesticides containing phosphorus, the MAK value of 0.2 mg/m^3 seems to include a sufficient safety margin." RR = 0.2/1.24 = 0.16. (MAK 1996: 0.2 mg/m^3)

Chloroacetic acid methyl ester is a colorless liquid that is used as a solvent and as an intermediate in chemical synthesis.
In 1993, the commission wrote: "After 28 days of exposure, the NOEL for the irritative effect was determined at 10 ppm (about 45 mg/m^3). . . . Taking the predominant local irritative effects into account, the MAK value is set at 1 ppm (5 mg/m^3). This value should be seen as provisional, since thus far a 28 days study is all the information available on systemic toxicty." RR = 1/10 = 0.10. (MAK 1996: 1 ppm)

In the following three cases, the MAK was based on an oral NOEL from animal experiments, hence requiring both an interspecies extrapolation and a route extrapolation. These cases are also included in Figure 3.2 and marked ''oral.''

Atrazine is a crystalline compound that is used as an herbicide. In its report (1981), the commission noted that a NOEL of 3.75 mg/kg had been determined in dogs. "According to Zielhaus's account, a safety factor of 10 (extrapolation from oral animal experiments to air concentrations) is sufficient for the situation on the workplace. Under the assumption of complete resorption of atrazine through the lungs, 0.375 mg/kg would correspond to a concentration in the air of 2.5 mg/m^3, i.e., a worker weighing 60 kg would in 8 hours inhale 9 m^3 air with this concentration of atrazine, and through this he would absorb 22.5 mg atrazine (= 0.375 mg/kg). A MAK value of 2.0 mg/m^3 seems, based on the available results, to provide sufficient safety..." A MAK of 2.0 mg/m^3 was chosen. RR = 0.08. (MAK 1996: 2.0 mg/m^3)

2,4-D is a yellow powder that is used as an herbicide. It was also one of the components of Agent Orange, which was used by the United States in the Vietnam War as a defoliant (a substance that causes leaves to drop off).
 The commission reported in 1994 that the oral NOEL in dogs was 0.3 mg/kg. "This value corresponds to an absorbed amount of about 21 mg for humans, corresponding to an exposure limit of 2 mg/m^3 if the inhaled air during a workshift amounts to 10 m^3. Due to the uncertainty of the extrapolation of a NOEL from oral administration to inhalation the MAK is lowered to 1 mg/m^3." RR = 1/2 = 0.50. (MAK 1996: 1 mg/m^3)

2,4,5-T is an herbicide and another ingredient in Agent Orange.
 In 1995, the commission wrote: "Based on the NOEL 2.4 mg/kg bodyweight in dogs, a concentration without effect of 17 mg/m^3 can be inferred for a human weighing 70 kg and inhaling 10 m^3 each workshift. Therefore the already established MAK value of 10 mg/m^3 is regarded as sufficient." RR = 10/17 = 0.59. (MAK 1996: 10 mg/m^3)

Hence, whereas the 1981 report on atrazine refers to the ''safety factor'' of 10 proposed by Zielhuis and van der Kreek (1979), much smaller margins were chosen in the reports on 2,4-D in 1994 and on 2,4,5-T in 1995. No explanation for this change in regulatory practice can be found in the published documentation.

As Figure 3.2 shows, the regulatory ratios vary between 0.08 and 1.00 for these substances. In 7 of the 16 cases, the regulatory ratio was 0.49 or higher (corresponding to "safety factors" ≤ 2). Since interspecies differences are often larger than a factor of 2, it must be expected that a substantial proportion of the MAKs obtained this way do not protect against adverse health effects.

Three cases when a MAK was based on an animal NOEL have not been included in Figure 3.2 since specific information about interspecies differences was used for the extrapolation. One of these cases is a report on 2-butoxyethanol (1982). Hemolytic effects had been shown in rats at 77 ppm but not at 25 ppm. The commission said: "Taking into account the fact that the haemolytic effects of the substance are weaker in man, it may be concluded that exposure to 20 ppm would not be expected to have adverse effects on health and includes a sufficient safety margin as long as skin contact with the substance is avoided."

The second case is a report on ethyl acrylate (1986). The NOEL for irritative lesions of the nasal epithelia of rats and mice was 5 ppm. The commission said: "Since the specific respiratory physiology of rodents (obligate nose breathers) results in increased local sensitivity, a MAK value of 5 ppm must be considered to be low enough to protect exposed humans from irritative damage to the respiratory passages."[10]

The third case is a report on diethylene glycol (1995). No results from chronic exposure of humans were available. Since "experiences from cases of [acute] intoxication show a sensitivity about 10 times higher than in animals, there are reasons to choose a safety margin of 10 with respect to the NOEL of the chronic animal experiments." The MAK was set at 10 ppm and was reported to correspond to 6 mg/kg under the assumption of 100% resorption. The lowest oral NOEL was 50 mg/kg (rat). Hence, the regulatory ratio was 6/50 = 0.12. Since humans were reported to be about 10 times more sensitive than the experimental animals, this means that no safety margin at all was considered necessary to compensate for possible errors.

ANIMAL EFFECT LEVELS

When a MAK is based on effect levels from animal experiments, two extrapolations are combined: from effect level to no-effect level and from laboratory animals to humans. Such combined extrapolations, based on inhalation experiments, were the basis for MAKs in the following 12 cases, which are summarized in Figure 3.3:

Chlorine is a gas that is used as a bleaching agent, a disinfectant, and a raw material in chemical synthesis.

In 1970, the MAK was set at 0.5 ppm to avoid "the subjective irritative effects in humans." It made use of data on "toxic-inflammatory changes in the airways of animals," namely, two experiments in which 0.7–1.7 ppm, in chronic exposure of rabbits, led to "clear changes in the lungs." RR = 0.5/0.7 = 0.71. (MAK 1996: 0.5 ppm)

p-Dichlorobenzene is a white crystalline substance that is used as an insecticide and a fumigant.

In 1991, the MAK was reduced to 50 ppm since studies in rats and mice had shown "slight changes in organ weights without histopathological findings" at 75 ppm. RR = 50/75 = 0.67. (MAK 1996: 50 ppm)

1,1,2-Trichloro-1,2,2-trifluoroethane is a colorless liquid (a Freon). Its major uses are as a refrigerant, a solvent, a degreasing agent, and an intermediate in chemical synthesis.

The commission wrote in 1988: "The data of Vainio et al reveal measurable hepatic effects after exposure to 1,1,2-trichloro-1,2,2-trifluoroethane concentrations at the level of the previous MAK value, 1000 ppm (minimum effect level). Although the relevance for man of these effects seen in experiments with rats (proliferation of the endoplasmic reticulum) is unclear, they did make it necessary to reconsider this very high MAK value." The MAK was reduced to 500 ppm. RR = 500/1000 = 0.50. (MAK 1996: 500 ppm)

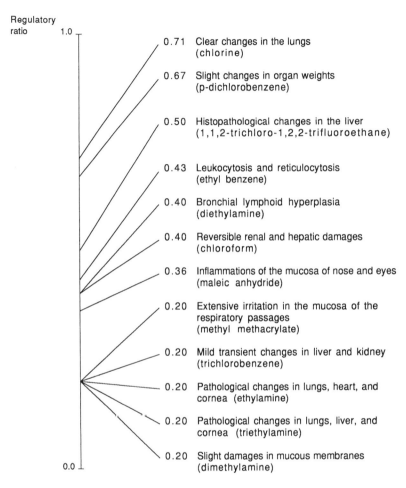

FIGURE 3.3. Regulatory ratios for MAKs based on animal effect levels. The effect levels all refer to respiratory exposure.

Ethyl benzene is a colorless liquid that is used in the rubber and plastics industries.

In 1985, the commission reported that in rodents, 230 ppm administered 4 hours a day for 7 months gave rise to "blood count changes in the form of leukocytosis and reticulocytosis.... Against this background, a MAK value of 100 ppm should be seen as provisional with respect to organ and blood status." RR = 100/230 = 0.43. (MAK 1996: 100 ppm)

Diethylamine is an unusually flammable liquid that is used in the chemical and rubber industries.

The commission wrote in 1984: "Lynch and coworkers found in rats, after 120 days' exposure to 25 ppm diethylamine, only an increase in the frequency of bronchial lymphoid hyperplasia. No 'no effect level' was found. Applying a reasonable safety margin, the MAK value is set at 10 ppm." RR = 10/25 = 0.40. (MAK 1996: 5 ppm)

Chloroform is a volatile colorless liquid that was previously used as an anesthetic. It is still used as a solvent and a raw material in chemical synthesis.

In 1976, an earlier MAK of 50 ppm was reduced to 10 ppm due to an experimental study in which 25 ppm gave rise to "slight, reversible renal and hepatic damages." RR = 10/25 = 0.40. (MAK 1996: 10 ppm)

Maleic anhydride is a white, crystalline solid and a raw material in the plastics and chemicals industries.

According to the commission's report (1990), at exposure to 1.1 mg/m^3 (0.27 ppm) "in primates, inflammation develops in the mucosa of nose and eyes but histological examination reveals minimal focal lesions.... The minimal findings in primates indicate that a MAK value of 0.1 ppm (0.4 mg/m^3) can provide sufficient protection for man." RR = 0.4/1.1 = 0.36. (MAK 1996: 0.1 ppm)

Methyl methacrylate is a colorless liquid that is used in the production of clear (glass-like) plastics.

In 1988, the MAK was reduced from 100 to 50 ppm because there was "only little difference between the unambiguously toxic concentration which produced extensive irritation in the mucosa of the respiratory passages of female rats (250 ppm)" and the previous MAK of 100 ppm. RR = 50/250 = 0.20. (MAK 1996: 50 ppm)

Trichlorobenzene is a colorless liquid that is used as a solvent and an insecticide, as well as in chemical synthesis.

The commission wrote in 1990: "In animal studies with the rat, which has been shown to be a relatively sensitive species, long-term inhalation of concentrations as low as 25 ppm induces mild transient changes in liver and kidney. For this reason a MAK value of 5 ppm has been suggested." This value was adopted. RR = 5/25 = 0.20. (MAK 1996: 5 ppm)

Ethylamine is a liquid or gas (it boils at 17 °C, 62 °F) that is used in the rubber and dyestuffs industries.

According to a 1984 report, the MAK of 10 ppm was based on "clear toxic findings at 50 ppm in animal experiments" involving rabbits. "At 50 ppm findings included peribronchitis, pneumonia, and thickening of the walls of small pulmonary vessels, to some extent also focal muscular degeneration of the heart. After 2 weeks of exposure to ethylamine at 50 ppm rabbits had multiple punctate erosions of the corneal epithelium, corneal edema, and edema of the nictitating membrane." RR = 10/50 = 0.20. (MAK 1996: 5 ppm)

Triethylamine is a colorless liquid that is used in the manufacture of plastics, as an anticorrosive agent, and in chemical synthesis.

In 1983, the commission wrote: "With respect to the unambiguous pathological changes in animal experiments that were observed at 50 ppm, the MAK is reduced to 10 ppm." The effects found at 50 ppm included slight thickening of vascular walls in the lungs, slight parenchymatous degeneration of the liver, and multiple punctate erosions of the corneal epithelium (Brieger and Hodes 1951). RR = 10/50 = 0.20. (MAK 1996: 1 ppm)

Dimethylamine is a gas but is often delivered in a water solution. It is used in the rubber and textiles industries.

The commission reported in 1993: "Since concentrations below 10 ppm have not been tried in 2-year studies, but 10 ppm in rats provoked slight damages in mucous membranes, the MAK is lowered to 2 ppm." The damages referred to had been found in the nasal epithelia of the animals. RR = 2/10 = 0.20. (MAK 1996: 2 ppm)

The regulatory ratios recorded in Figure 3.3 range between 0.20 and 0.71. No clear correlation can be found between the regulatory ratios and the severity of the pertinent effects.

One would expect these ratios to be much lower than those in Figure 3.2 since effect levels require one more extrapolation step than no-effect levels. However, the geometric mean of the values in Figure 3.2 is 0.33, and that of the values in Figure 3.3 is also 0.33. These findings indicate that the MAK commission may not have paid sufficient attention to the crucial distinction between effect levels and NOELs.

Two MAKs that have been determined on the basis of animal-effect levels were not included in Figure 3.3, since the commission referred to specific differences in susceptibility between humans and experimental animals. In both of these cases, they referred to the obligate nose breathing of rodents, and in one of them to strain-specific properties of the lachrimal gland as well:

Methyl acrylate is a colorless liquid that is used primarily in the production of acrylic fibers.

The commission wrote in 1985: "The only substance-related effects of a 2-year exposure to a concentration of 15 ppm were slight changes caused by irritation in a highly localized area of the nasal cavity and corneal changes. The corneal findings are a result of the specific age-related changes in the lacrimal glands of the strain of rat that was used and cannot be extrapolated directly to man. The specific respiratory physiology of the rat (obligate nose breathing) results in high local sensitivity of this species so that a MAK value of 5 ppm provides sufficient protection for man." RR = 5/15 = 0.33. (MAK 1996: 5 ppm)

n-Butyl acrylate is a colorless liquid that is used in paints and in the manufacture of fibers.

The commission wrote in 1985: "Inhalation of a butyl acrylate concentration of 15 ppm for 2 years caused only slight irritation of a highly localized area in the nasal cavity. The specific respiratory physiology of the rat (obligate nose breathing) leads to high local sensitivity in this species so that a MAK value of 10 ppm may be considered to ensure adequate protection for the human respiratory passages." RR = 10/15 = 0.67. (MAK 1996: 2 ppm)

As we saw above (in the section on "Animal No-Effect Levels"), a similar argument was applied to ethyl acrylate (1986). For that substance, a no-effect level in rodents for nasal irritation was chosen as a MAK. However, in a more recent report on dimethylamine (1993; see above and Figure 3.3), slight damage of the nasal epithelia in rats and mice at 10 ppm was the reason for a reduction of the MAK to 2 ppm. No reason was given for this difference in practice.

Since nose breathing protects the lungs, the smaller risk of nasal damage in humans exposed to these substances may be accompanied by a larger risk of damage to bronchial and pulmonary epithelia. No discussion of this eventuality was found in the documentation reports.

ON NOT LEARNING FROM EXPERIENCE

We have now tested the hypothesis (HC4) that the regulatory ratios are approximately the same for substances that have the same critical effects and the same types of reference levels. This hypothesis proved to be false: The regulatory ratios were found to vary widely in a way that does not correlate with the severity of the critical effect. These findings speak against the more basic hypothesis that the MAKs are based exclusively on health criteria.

As can be seen in Figures 3.1–3.3, many regulatory ratios are about 0.5 or higher (corresponding to safety factors of 2 or less). With such small margins of safety, it must be expected that a substantial proportion of the MAKs do not protect against adverse health effects.

The commission itself provided an illustrative example of this problem in its report on *n*-hexane (1982). This substance had its MAK reduced in 1974 from 500 to 100 ppm "because long-term occupational exposure to 400 ppm or more was known at that time to lead to polyneuritis." Hence, a safety factor of 4 seems to have been applied.

Later, this MAK was shown to be inadequate since "neurotoxic effects first appear in animals exposed to concentrations above 200 ppm whereas the human organism can react with polyneuropathic symptoms at as little as 100 ppm." It was concluded that the previous MAK value of 100 ppm "cannot ensure adequate health protection for employees," and the MAK was reduced to 50 ppm. Hence, in spite of the failure of the previous safety factor of 4, this time a factor of only 2 was chosen.

The commission has accumulated abundant experience showing that the safety factors it usually applies are insufficient, so that subsequent reductions of the MAKs are often required. However, it does not seem to have concluded from this experience that larger safety factors should be introduced. It is difficult to understand the reason if the protection of health was the only consideration.

STANDARDS OF EVIDENCE

The documentation reports were also searched for cases in which particularly weak evidence was accepted as the basis for MAKs. Probably the weakest evidence on which MAKs have been based can be found in two early reports in which the absence of information about a certain type of effect in exposed humans was taken as sufficient evidence that such an effect does not exist.

The first of these is the document on p-benzoquinone (1970). Here the commission mentioned a 4 month study in rats showing thrombocytopenia at 0.06–0.08 ppm. They also referred to a field study that showed both anemia and thrombocytopenia among workers exposed to 0.02–0.08 ppm. However, in their summary, the commission put this information aside:

> Considering the experiments with chronic inhalation and the field experiences ... the MAK of 0.1 ppm seems relatively high. On the other hand, when this value has been complied with in some other countries for about 30 years, systemic effects have not been observed. The now valid value

0.1 ppm is therefore retained, with reference being made to the necessity to avoid any skin contact with *p*-benzoquinone.

No reference was given for the lack of negative effects in "some other countries," nor were these countries even identified. Hence the MAK was based on the *absence* of known reports of such effects from other countries. In view of the fact that many serious health effects have gone unreported for decades, this can hardly be called a scientifically sound argument.

The second case is a report on malathion (1972). The commission mentioned four inhalation experiments in animals. One of these showed a level of 67.5 mg/m^3 to be without toxic effects, whereas the other three showed toxic effects at much lower levels (2.26, 1.2, and 0.075 mg/m^3, respectively). The commission concluded:

> Quite diverging concentration limits for toxicity were found in subacute and chronic inhalation experiments with animals. These concentrations were partly clearly above, partly also below the MAK value of 15 mg/m^3. In spite of these differences, the MAK value that has been valid for more than 10 years seems to be sufficiently safe, since no cases of intoxication have been made known from production and use of malathion in large quantities.

Again, no documentation was given for this absence of cases of intoxication, and again the mere absence of reports from human exposure was allowed to take precedence over worrisome reports from animal experiments.

The MAK for *p*-benzoquinone is still (1996) 0.1 ppm, and that for malathion is still 15 mg/m^3. Hence, the arguments on which these MAKs were based still have regulatory impact. (No similar arguments were found in later documentation reports.)

In more recent reports, the quality of NOELs is a more pertinent issue. The quality of a NOEL depends on both biological and statistical factors. From a biological point of view, a NOEL based on the most susceptible of several tested species and strains offers more reliable protection than one based on a single species and strain. If metabolic

68　SETTING THE LIMIT

information is available, strains that metabolize the substance in the same way as humans should have been tested. From a statistical point of view, it is essential that the animal groups not be too small.

In its report on cyclohexane (1971), the commission claimed that "[t]he harmless concentration of cyclohexane for rabbits" was between 435 and 786 ppm. This conclusion was based on a single experiment with only eight rabbits (Treon et al. 1943). In later years, NOELs based on a single experiment with 10 animals were accepted as a standard, as in the following examples:

2-Methoxyethanol is a colorless liquid that has multiple uses as an industrial solvent.

In the commission's 1982 report on this substance, the NOEL for testis damage was said to be about 30 ppm. This conclusion was based on one experiment in which 10 male rabbits were exposed to 30 ppm for 6–7 months and no toxic effects on the testicles were found. (One more experiment with rabbits exposed to 30 ppm was mentioned. In that study, degenerative changes in the testicular epithelium were discovered in one of five rabbits after 3 months' exposure.) The same statement, based on the same information, was repeated in a new report on the same substance (1992).

Chloroacetic acid methyl ester is a colorless liquid that is used as a solvent and as an intermediate in chemical synthesis.

In the commission's report on this substance (1993), the NOEL for irritative effects was taken to be 10 ppm, based on one study in which 10 rats had been exposed to that concentration.

Ten animals is a small group for the determination of NOELs. If an effect has a true frequency of 7% under experimental conditions, then the probability that it will not appear in a test on ten animals is 48%. Even if the true frequency is as high as 25%, the probability that it will not be seen in a test on ten animals is as high as 6%.

A similar overinterpretation of a negative result can be found in a report on vinylidene chloride.

Vinylidene chloride (VDC) is a colorless liquid that is used primarily in the production of plastics.

Reporting on this substance (1985), the commission noted that the most sensitive animal strain was Swiss mice. In their summary, they said: "In only one single inhalation study with Swiss mice was 25 ppm VDC associated with chronic-toxic hepatic and renal damages and with an increased number of renal adenocarcinomas, in particular in male mice. At 50 ppm the inhalation had to be interrupted after 4 exposures due to high mortality; and an adenocarcinoma was found among the surviving animals in this group. In this study, chronic inhalation of 10 ppm was tolerated by Swiss mice without hepatic or renal damage. No renal carcinomas were found in this [10 ppm] group."

This passage creates the impression that the study referred to gives us reasons to believe that although 25 ppm causes cancer in these animals, 10 ppm does not. A simple statistical analysis of the published data shows that this is not so. In this experiment, tumors appeared in 28 of 119 male animals exposed to 25 ppm and in none of 24 male animals exposed to 10 ppm. For an experiment to refute the hypothesis that the substance causes tumors at 10 ppm as well as at 25 ppm, it must refute the simple linear hypothesis that the frequency of tumors at 10 ppm is 10/25 that at 25 ppm. According to that hypothesis, the frequency of tumors among animals exposed to 10 ppm is $(28/119) \times (10/25) = 0.094$. Given this, the probability of the result obtained (that is, of no tumors among 24 animals at 10 ppm) is 0.09. Hence, the outcome of this experiment does not deviate significantly from the linear hypothesis, and consequently it does not support the conclusion that this substance does not cause cancer in Swiss mice at 10 ppm. (It should perhaps be mentioned that later in 1985, Maltoni and coworkers [1985,

p. 43] reported that 10 ppm of vinylidene chloride gave rise to lung tumors and mammary adenocarcinomas in Swiss mice.)

QUESTIONABLE REPORTING

No systematic study was made of the accuracy of the commission's summaries from the scientific literature, but four questionable cases were discovered. In two of these, a concentration at which an effect is manifest was mentioned in a way that created the erroneous impression that this was the lowest concentration associated with the effect.

Trichloroethylene is a solvent and a degreasing agent.

In 1976, the commission referred to the fact that 6 years earlier, it had "reduced the MAK to 50 ppm. Decisive for this were results of field investigations and studies by commission members, according to which, at average concentrations of trichloroethylene (over the working week) of 100 ppm disturbances of the central nervous system were observed in the form of a so-called 'psycho-organic syndrome' with neurological impairments and psychological changes as well as visual disturbances."

Four references were given to substantiate these effects at 100 ppm. One was unpublished. Three were articles in the medical literature: (1) Takamatsu (1962) reported subjective symptoms as well as visual disturbances at 50–100 ppm, whereas no such effects appeared in a group of 14–16 workers exposed below 50 ppm. (2) Andersson (1957, esp. pp. 55–57, 153) reported neurasthenic symptoms among about 40% of workers with <20 mg/liter trichloroacetic acid in urine, 60% with 20–75 mg/liter and 80% at >75 mg/liter. According to Andersson, 75 mg/liter corresponds, to about 30 ppm. (3) Grandjean and coworkers (1955) reported that symptoms of chronic poisoning, including neurological and psychological symptoms, were caused by "exposure to concentrations of tri in the air varying, in general, between 20 and 80 p.p.m.[,] the average being about 40 p.p.m." Hence, the published sources referred to by the commission revealed neurological and psychological disturbances at levels far *below* 100 ppm.

Ethylene chlorohydrin is a colorless liquid that is used as a solvent and a raw material for chemical synthesis.

In the summary of its report on this substance (1983), the commission said that analogies with related substances indicated that 5 ppm would be a reasonable MAK. "On the other hand, some few individual observations suggest that particular caution is necessary. It is repeated here that, although the concentration data must be considered questionable, inhalation of 18 ppm has resulted in marked symptoms of intoxication in man and that exposure to 7.5 and 32 ppm was lethal for rats. Because of this remaining uncertainty, the MAK value is set at 1 ppm."

This text gives the impression that 7.5 ppm was the lowest lethal concentration in the experiment referred to. This was not the case. The summary of the original report says: "Only a small concentration in the inhaled air, 7.5 p.p.m., for one hour was required to cause death. A concentration of 4 p.p.m. was not fatal if the exposure was limited to one hour; on a second exposure after two hours it was as fatal as 7.5 p.p.m. A concentration of 2 p.p.m. was not fatal on a single exposure; however, with repeated exposure this concentration caused paralysis in some rats and finally death" (Ambrose 1950, p. 596).

In two cases, what was actually an average concentration was referred to as the lower limit of a range of concentrations.

Xylene is a colorless liquid that is present in gasoline and in petroleum solvents, as well as in many solvent-based products such as paints.

In 1983, the commission wrote: "Since the vestibule of the ear is known to be disturbed under exposure to xylene concentrations between 90 and 280 ppm, it is strongly suspected that the now valid MAK of 200 ppm is too high. It is therefore lowered to 100 ppm."

This passage creates the impression that these effects were found in conditions with concentrations fluctuating between the extreme values 90 and 280 ppm. In fact, they were found in exposure chambers at various average levels, one of which was 90 ppm. In their summary, the authors of the cited article emphasized that "psychophysiological functions, such as reaction time, manual coordination and body balance" were impaired at 90 ppm (Savolainen et al. 1980).

2,4,6-Trinitrotoluene (TNT) is a colorless or yellow crystalline substance that is used primarily as an explosive.

In the commission's 1988 report, a study by Savolainen and coworkers was summarized as follows: "Cataract formation has been observed after prolonged exposure to 0.1–0.35 mg/m^3." This statement gives the impression that the concentration fluctuated between the extreme values 0.1 and 0.35 mg/m^3. (The MAK in 1996 is 0.09 mg/m^3.)

In fact, the study included two groups of workers: five men exposed to an average of 0.35 mg/m^3 (range, 0.31–0.39) and four men exposed to an average of 0.10 mg/m^3 (range, 0.02–0.19). All four workers in the latter group had binocular cataracts that the researchers considered to have been caused by TNT exposure (Savolainen et al. 1985).

CONCLUSIONS

The documentation reports underlying the MAKs are comprehensive and qualified summaries of the toxicological literature on the respective substances. In general, they give a reliable picture of the known risks associated with exposure to the substances. On the other hand, the uncertainties involved are not much discussed.

The MAKs share with the TLVs the important advantage of being updated yearly. The German legal system is clearly more efficient in this respect than the American one, in which OSHA's attempts to update exposure limits have been blocked by litigation.

However, the MAKs do not fulfill the promise of being purely health-based. We have seen numerous examples of how MAKs have been influenced by other factors. Many MAKs have been established at about half the value at which an unwanted effect is known to appear in humans or at about half of the lowest value with no adverse effects in animals. The commission has repeatedly found that such "safety factors" were too small, and MAKs had to be reduced further. It does not seem to have drawn the obvious conclusion that larger safety margins are needed to protect human health.

Since neither TLVs nor MAKs offer reliable protection of workers' health, we now turn to the Swedish exposure limits, which appear to be the lowest in the Western world. Are they sufficiently protective?

4

THE LOWEST VALUES

As we saw in Chapter 1, the Swedish occupational exposure limits are lower than those of other Western countries. Furthermore, in Sweden an ambitious attempt has been made to separate the scientific issues from the wider policy issues. Since 1978, the two types of issues have been managed by two different committees.

THE DEVELOPMENT OF SWEDISH EXPOSURE LIMITS

Official lists of exposure limits for chemicals in Sweden are issued by the National Board of Occupational Safety and Health. The first list, published in 1969, was based almost entirely on the TLVs of the ACGIH. The second list was issued in 1974 and took effect in 1975. No documentation for these two lists was published. Partly in response to criticism of the lack of documentation, a new procedure for the determination of OELs was introduced in 1978. Since then, two working groups have been involved in the process: the Criteria Group and the Regulations Group.

The Criteria Group consists of scientists in the relevant fields. Its task is to gather and evaluate the available scientific and medical information on substances that the Regulations Group selects for its consideration. Its findings are summarized in consensus reports of 5–15 pages, which are published in both English and Swedish. Many of these reports are based on much longer and more detailed criteria documents, some of which have been commissioned by the Criteria Group itself. The Criteria Group bases its conclusions on the evidence available in the scientific literature. Unpublished information, e.g., from industry, is not taken into account (Rudén 1997). The group does not have resources for commissioning new epidemiological or experimental studies.

Whenever possible, the Criteria Group identifies a critical effect and reports a dose–response relationship. It does *not* propose an OEL. Instead, this is done by the Regulations Group, using the information from the Criteria Group and information on technological and economical feasibility (Lundberg and Holmberg 1985; Nordberg et al. 1988; Lundberg et al. 1991).

Table 4.1 and Figure 4.1 show the development of the overall level of Swedish OELs for all substances, for substances classified as carcinogens, and for solvents. The overall change for all substances from 1969 to 1994 corresponds to an average yearly reduction by 3.9%. (It can also be expressed as a "half-life" for OELs of 17 years.) Most of this change took place during the first 10 years. From 1969 to 1979, the average yearly reduction was 6.3%, and from 1979 to 1994 it was only 2.2%. Hence, perhaps surprisingly, the rate of reduction slowed down substantially after the establishment of the Criteria Group in 1978.

For carcinogens, the rate of reduction was much higher than for substances in general. The average yearly reduction for carcinogens from 1969 to 1994 was 10% (corresponding to a "half-life" of 7

TABLE 4–1. Overall Changes in Swedish OELs

YEAR	AVERAGE LEVEL COMPARED TO 1969		
	ALL SUBSTANCES	CARCINOGENS	SOLVENTS
1969	1.00	1.00	1.00
1975	0.63	0.27	0.76
1979	0.52	0.14	0.58
1982	0.49	0.13	0.52
1985	0.46	0.12	0.46
1988	0.44	0.11	0.42
1990	0.41	0.10	0.36
1991	0.40	0.09	0.32
1994	0.37	0.08	0.28

Geometric means and the adjacent-list method have been used (see the Appendix).

The column for carcinogens contains substances that were classified as carcinogens in 1994. (There were 33 such substances with OELs in 1994. Thirteen of them had OELs in 1969, 19 in 1975, 29 in 1979, 31 in 1982–1985, and 32 in 1988–1991.)

The column for solvents contains substances that are included in De Renzo's list of solvents (De Renzo 1986) but that were not classified as carcinogens in the 1994 list of OELs. (There were 24 of these substances in 1969, 32 in 1975, 56 in 1979, 60 in 1982, 72 in 1985, 78 in 1988 and 1990, 82 in 1991, and 95 in 1994.)

years). For solvents, the average yearly reduction was 5.0%, only slightly more than for all substances.

To investigate the relationship of Swedish OELs to the TLVs, the values on each of the nine Swedish lists were tabulated against the corresponding TLV values in force at the time it was issued. In 1969, 79% of the Swedish values coincided with the TLVs, and in 1975, 57%. After that, between 48% and 52% of the values on the Swedish lists of OELs coincided with the TLVs. In most cases, when the two lists differed, the Swedish list had the lower value. In 1994, 48% of the values on the Swedish list coincided with the TLVs, 9% were higher, and 43% were lower.

The geometric means of the quotients between Swedish OELs and

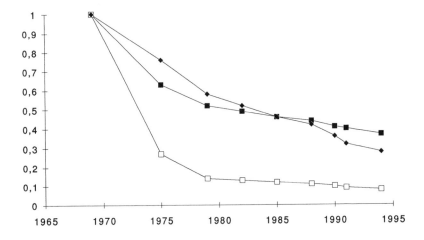

- All substances
- Carcinogens
- Solvents

FIGURE 4.1. Development of the overall level of the Swedish OELs. For details, see Table 4.1 and the Appendix.

the TLVs of the ACGIH are reported in Table 4.2 and Figure 4.2. After a remarkable reduction from 0.91 to 0.62 in 1975, the mean quotient rose to 0.71 in 1982, a value that (after some minor fluctuations) still stands. For carcinogens, the corresponding quotient is much lower, 0.35. These statistics confirm that carcinogenicity is more strictly treated by Swedish authorities than by the ACGIH.

THE IMPACT OF CONSENSUS REPORTS

Consensus reports are produced by the Criteria Group both to determine OELs for new substances and to reconsider existing OELs. The use of consensus reports for the latter purpose is summarized in Table 4.3. As

TABLE 4–2. Geometric Means of the OEL/TLV Quotients for the Swedish List of OELs

YEAR	MEAN OEL/TLV QUOTIENT		
	ALL SUBSTANCES	CARCINOGENS	SOLVENTS
1969	0.91	0.88	1.01
1975	0.62	0.35	0.80
1979	0.59	0.23	0.72
1982	0.71	0.32	0.84
1985	0.73	0.35	0.86
1988	0.73	0.37	0.80
1990	0.67	0.28	0.70
1991	0.65	0.27	0.67
1994	0.70	0.35	0.68

Carcinogens and solvents are defined as in Table 4.1.

the table shows, when the list of OELs for 1988 was adopted, there were 41 new reports from the Criteria Group on substances that already had OELs. ("New" means that these reports were not available on the day when the preceding list of OELs was adopted.) Only three of these values were changed.

Over the whole period, 29 of the 148 decisions (20%) for which a new consensus report was available led to a change in the OEL (28 decreases and 1 increase). More important, of the 106 changes in OELs during this period, 29 (27%) took place when a new consensus report was available. No doubt, information not reported in a consensus report may provide legitimate grounds for changes in OELs. On the other hand, it is incontestably a desideratum that a new consensus report should be available when an OEL is reconsidered by the Regulations Group. The fact that this was the case for only 27% of the decisions that led to a revised value indicates that the coordination between the Consensus Group and the Regulations Group can be improved.

On the other hand, the availability of a new consensus report can be shown to be associated with greater reductions in OELs. Over the period when the system with consensus reports was operative (1982–

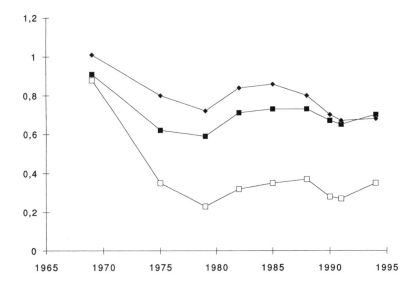

FIGURE 4.2. Development of the OEL/TLV quotients. For details, see Table 4.2.

1994), the geometric mean of the ratio between new and previous OELs was 0.85 for substances with a new consensus report.[1] The corresponding mean for all substances was 0.95.

Over the whole period from 1979 to mid-1993 (when the list for 1994 was decided), the Criteria Group produced 148 consensus reports on substances that already had an OEL. This corresponds to an average annual output of about 10–11 reappraisals. At the same time, about ten new OELs were introduced every year.[2] It should also be noted that some substances have been reappraised more than once. Hence, at the present publication rates of new OELs and of reappraisal reports, a regular science-based revision of all Swedish OELs cannot be achieved.

TABLE 4–3. Changes in OELs for Which a New Consensus Report Was Available

	1982	1985	1988	1990	1991	1994	SUM
Number of OELs for which a new consensus report was available	19	47	41	12	10	19	148
Number of these with a changed OEL	2	15	3	1	2	6	29
Total number of changed OELs	17	19	14	26	12	18	106

CRITICAL EFFECTS

Whenever the Criteria Group finds it possible to identify a critical effect, it does so. The *critical effect* is the adverse effect that appears at the lowest exposure level (Nordberg et al. 1988). The idea is that by protecting against the critical effect, an exposure limit should also protect against all other adverse effects. The Criteria Group also attempts to provide as reliable information as possible about the dose–response relationship for the critical effect.

To investigate how this information about critical effects and their dose–response relationships has influenced the Swedish OELs, the relevant information was extracted from the consensus reports and compared to the latest list of exposure limits. The consensus reports are available in 15 printed volumes in the *Arbete och Hälsa* series and add up to 1735 pages.[3] In each of these reports, the critical effect and the dose-related information pertaining to the critical effect were sought. Hence, if a substance was assigned decreased lung function as its critical effect, the consensus report was searched for dose-related information referring to decreased lung function.

Only information based on experience from human subjects was included in the analysis. (Exceptions to this rule were made in the few cases in which the Criteria Group made it clear that it considered dose-related information from animal experiments to be directly relevant to humans.) Hence, unless otherwise stated, all information about effects at various exposure levels referred to in this chapter is based on experience in humans. Studies on human subjects that the Criteria Group considered to be unreliable were excluded from consideration.

The dose-related information given in the consensus reports was divided into four categories. (*1*) For some substances, the committee specified one or more levels at which the critical effect does not appear. The highest such level was called a *no-effect level* (NEL) for the critical effect. (*2*) In some cases, the committee reported a "threshold" below which the critical effect will not appear, but without stating whether or not the effect is present at the threshold value itself. Such levels were recorded as *threshold levels* (TL). (*3*) In other cases, the committee gave no NEL or TL but instead reported concentrations at which the critical effect *does* appear. The lowest such level mentioned in the report was called the *effect level* (EL) for the critical effect. (*4*) For a few substances (mostly carcinogens), more elaborate dose–response relations were reported.[4]

The NELs, TLs, and ELs were compared to the current Swedish list of OELs (ASS 1993). (These are time-weighted averages unless otherwise stated.) For a substance that has a NEL, the OEL/NEL ratio is defined in the obvious way as the quotient between the OEL and the NEL. OEL/TL and OEL/EL ratios are defined analogously. These are all variants of the regulatory ratios (RR) introduced in Chapter 3.

From 1979 to the first half of 1994, consensus reports for 278 substances were prepared by the Criteria Group.[5] For 63% of these substances, a critical effect was specified.[6] This includes the many cases in which the critical effect was reported only with reservations such as "probably" or "judging from animal experiments."

The number of substances with various types of critical effects are summarized in Table 4.4. For 13% of the substances, more than one critical effect was given. Among the remaining substances, by far the most common critical effect was irritation of the eyes and mucous membranes (41%), followed by respiratory diseases (15%), tumors (11%), effects on the central nervous system (6%), effects on blood and blood-forming or-

TABLE 4–4. Critical Effects Assigned in Consensus Reports

CRITICAL EFFECT	NUMBER OF SUBSTANCES
Irritation of eyes and mucous membranes	59
Effects on the respiratory system (other than irritation of upper passages)	22
Cancer (all tumors)	16
CNS effects	9
Effects on the blood and blood-forming organs	8
Effects on the liver	6
PNS effects (peripheral nervous system)	3
Genotoxicity	3
Odor	3
Embryotoxicity and teratogenicity	2
Taste	2
Effects on the eyes (other than irritation)	2
Effects on the heart and circulatory system	2
Effects on the kidney	2
Metal fume fever	1
Reproductive effects	1
Discoloration of tissues	1
Skin effects (other than irritation)	1
Effects on the thyroid	1
Multiple (several effects given as critical)	21

gans (6%), and liver disease (4%). In what follows, the regulatory ratios for the major effect groups will be studied in detail.

IRRITATION EFFECTS

Irritation of the eyes and mucous membranes was the critical effect assigned to no fewer than 59 substances. The dose–effect information that was available for these substances can be summarized as follows:

NEL	4	(7%)
TL	2	(3%)

| EL | 32 | (54%) |
| No information | 21 | (36%) |

NELs and TLs are adequate data for the determination of OELs that protect the exposed population. ELs are much less useful for that purpose. From the fact that, say, 25 ppm of a substance irritates the eyes, we cannot conclude at what levels that effect does *not* occur. Therefore, it is unfortunate that NELs or TLs were available only in 10% of the cases, and that in more than a third of the cases not even ELs were available.

The following six substances had an NEL or a TL:

Hydrogen sulfide is a gas that occurs in petroleum and in natural gas. It is also formed as a by-product in many chemical reactions involving sulphur compounds.

A consensus report in 1983 stated that 0.007 mg/m^3 "[i]n most cases causes no irritation" and that 15–30 mg/m^3 is a "threshold for eye irritation." Since the OEL is 14 mg/m^3, the latter value yields an OEL/TL ratio of 0.47–0.93.

Acetone is a colorless liquid that has many uses in the chemical industry, including the manufacture of plastics and paints.

A consensus report in 1987 stated that 300 ppm but not 200 ppm gives rise to irritation of the nose, throat, and eyes. The OEL is 250 ppm. Hence, the OEL/NEL ratio is 1.25.

Caprolactam is a white solid that is used primarily in the production of synthetic fibers.

According to a 1989 report, irritation effects do not appear below 32 mg/m^3 (but they do appear at 46–116 mg/m^3). The OEL is 5 mg/m^3, and hence the OEL/NEL ratio is 0.16.

Trimellitic anhydride is a white solid that is used in the production of plastics and paints.

A consensus report from 1989 gave a NEL of 0.1 mg/m^3. The OEL is 0.04 mg/m^3, and hence the OEL/NEL ratio is 0.4.

Maleic anhydride is a white, crystalline solid and a raw material in the plastics and chemicals industries.

In 1989 the committee said that "[t]he threshold for nasal irritation in human subjects has been reported to be 5.5 mg/m^3." (They also mentioned that 1.1 mg/m^3 "resulted in irritation in the noses and eyes of rats, hamsters and monkeys." Since they did not explicitly say that this value is relevant to humans, it will not be taken into account here.) The OEL is 1.2 mg/m^3, and the OEL/TL ratio is 0.22.

Dipropylene glycol monomethyl ether is a colorless liquid that is used as a solvent and as a constituent of cosmetic products.

In 1990, the committee said that "[t]he limit for irritation has been reported to be 450 mg/m^3 (74 ppm)."[7] The OEL is 300 mg/m^3 (50 ppm); hence the OEL/TL ratio is 0.67.

In summary, it was possible to calculate three OEL/NEL ratios (1.25, 0.16, and 0.4) and three OEL/TL ratios (0.47–0.93, 0.22, and 0.67) for irritants. The geometric mean of these six values is 0.42–0.47.

The 32 substances for which ELs (but not NELs or TLs) were given are listed in Table 4.5. In contrast to NELs and TLs, ELs offer no protection. Therefore, OEL/EL ratios should be on average much smaller than OEL/NEL or OEL/TL ratios, perhaps about one order of magnitude smaller. (In the determination of Allowable Daily Intakes, an extra factor of 10 is conventionally applied if the lowest experimental dose had significant adverse effects, so that a lowest observed adverse effect level has to be used instead of a no observed adverse effect level [Catalano and Ryan 1994; Pohl and Abadin 1995].)

Surprisingly enough, the geometric mean of the OEL/EL ratios in Table 4.5 is 0.47–0.58, which is slightly *higher* than the mean of the OEL/NEL and OEL/TL ratios calculated above (0.42–0.47). Based on this result, it can be questioned whether the Regulations Group has paid sufficient attention to the distinction between ELs and NELs. (In the section ''On Not Learning from Experience'' in Chapter 3, the same question was asked about the German MAK commission.)

To achieve full protection against irritation of eyes and mucous

TABLE 4–5. ELs for Irritation of Eyes and Mucous Membranes

SUBSTANCE, REPORT YEAR	EFFECT LEVEL (EL)	SWEDISH OEL	OEL/EL
Isopropanol (1981)	400 ppm	150 ppm	0.38
Ethylene glycol (1981)	140 mg/m^3	25 mg/m^3	0.18
1-Butanol (1981)	25 ppm	15 ppm	0.6
Formaldehyde (1982)	0.05 ppm	0.5 ppm	10
Cyclohexanone (1983)	50 ppm	25 ppm	0.5
Amyl acetate (1983)	200 ppm	100 ppm	0.5
Furfural (1984)	5–14 ppm	2 ppm	0.14–0.40
Hydrogen fluoride (1984)	1.3–4.2 mg/m^3	1.7 mg/m^3*	0.4–1.3
1-Butyl acetate (1984)	200–300 ppm	100 ppm	0.33–0.50
White spirit (1986)	220 mg/m^3	300 mg/m^3	1.36
1-Nitropropane (1986)	100 ppm	5 ppm	0.05
Propylene glycol monomethyl ether (1986)	100 ppm	50 ppm	0.5
Allyl alcohol (1986)	12–30 mg/m^3	5 mg/m^3	0.17–0.42
Acetaldehyde (1987)	50 ppm	25 ppm	0.5
Diacetone alcohol (1988)	475 mg/m^3	120 mg/m^3	0.25
Acetic acid (1988)	25 ppm	5 ppm	0.2
Grain dust (1988)	1 mg/m^3	—	—
Vinyl acetate (1989)	5 ppm	5 ppm	1.0
Phthalic anhydride (1989)	0.2 mg/m^3	2 mg/m^3	10
Hydrogen peroxide (1989)	7 ppm†	1 ppm	0.14
Methyl acetate (1990)	4050 ppm	150 ppm	0.04
Ethanol (1990)	2000 ppm	500 ppm	0.25
Ethyl acetate (1990)	720 mg/m^3	500 mg/m^3	0.69
Vinyl toluene (1990)	10 ppm†	10 ppm	1.0
Ammonia (1991)	35 mg/m^3	18 mg/m^3	0.51
Isophorone (1991)	25 ppm	5 ppm*	0.2
Dioxane (1992)	50 ppm	25 ppm	0.5
Methyl methacrylate (1993)	6.7–68 mg/m^3	200 mg/m^3	2.9–30
Ethyl ether (1993)	200 ppm	400 ppm	2.0
Hexylene glycol (1993)	50 ppm	—	—
Dicyclopentadiene (1994)	1 ppm	—	—
o-Chloro-bensylidene malonitrile (1994)	0.004 mg/m^3	—	—

*Ceiling value. †The values for hydrogen peroxide and vinyl toluene derive from animal experiments referred to in the Conclusions section of the respective consensus reports. All other ELs in the table are based on human experience.

membranes, much lower OELs seem to be required for many of the substances listed in Table 4.5. However, since the irritation effects recorded in the ELs vary in strength, different OEL/EL ratios would be required for different substances to achieve the same degree of protection. A closer look at four of the substances will illustrate the differences:

Acetic acid is a colorless liquid that is used as a raw material in synthesis and as a solvent in the chemicals and plastics industries. (Vinegar, the household product, is a 4–6% aqueous solution of acetic acid.)

A level of 25 ppm causes "extreme irritation of the eyes and nose" in unaccustomed persons, and 50 ppm "is considered unendurable." Since no lower exposure level with irritation effects is mentioned in the report, the EL was 25 ppm. The OEL is 5 ppm, and the OEL/EL ratio is 0.2.

Phthalic anhydride is a white crystalline solid. It is used in the manufacture of plastics and has many other uses in the chemicals industry.

"Eye irritation (conjunctivitis) and runny noses (rhinitis) . . . were noted in a group of 25 persons exposed to dust concentrations below 0.2 mg/m^3 for 0.3 to 40 years." The OEL is 2 mg/m^3, and the OEL/EL ratio is 10.

Vinyl acetate is a colorless liquid that is used in the production of (polyvinyl) plastics. It is also a component of latex paints.

"[A]verage concentrations of 5 to 10 ppm vinyl acetate seem to have no effect on most people. . . . A few cases of irritation have been reported at concentrations as low as 5 ppm." This has been interpreted as an EL of 5 ppm. The OEL is 5 ppm, and the OEL/EL ratio is 1.0.

Ethyl ether ("ether") is a colorless, volatile liquid that was previously used as an anesthetic. Today it is used primarily as a solvent in the chemical industry.

"Subjects in an exposure-chamber study reported that they began to feel irritation in the nose and throat after three to five minutes of exposure to 200 ppm (616 mg/m³)." Furthermore, "[m]ost of the subjects judged that it would be impossible to endure an 8-hour workday at an exposure of 300 ppm (924 mg/m³)." This has been interpreted as an EL of 200 ppm. Since the OEL is 400 ppm, the OEL/EL ratio is 2.0.

An OEL at a fifth of a level that gives rise to "extreme irritation" (acetic acid) may very well be less protective than one at the exact level that gives rise to irritation in "a few cases" (vinyl acetate). Hence, an OEL/EL ratio of 0.2 may be less protective than one of 1.0 due to the different natures of the ELs. Because of the lack of dose-related information on the strength of irritation effects, no meaningful statistics based on such gradations could be made.

For none of the 28 substances with OELs in Table 4.5 does the consensus report allow the conclusion that the present Swedish OEL offers full protection against its assigned critical effect. For seven of them (namely, those with an OEL/EL ratio ≥ 1.0), it indicates that such protection is not obtained.

RESPIRATORY DISEASES

Disturbances of the respiratory organs (except for irritation of the upper passages) were indicated as critical effects in 22 consensus reports. Diisocyanates were treated in two reports (1982 and 1988), the second of which will be discussed here. For 6 of the 21 substances, no information on dose–effect relationships was available.[8] For 3 substances, an NEL can be deduced from the consensus report and for 12 an EL.

The three substances with NELs are listed in Table 4.6. For two of these substances the NEL protects against asthma and for one against pulmonary fibrosis. The geometric mean of their OEL/NEL ratios is ≥ 1.4. This value is surprisingly high compared to the mean of the six OEL/NEL and OEL/TL ratios for irritation effects reported above (0.42–0.47). Pulmonary fibrosis and asthma are more serious health

TABLE 4–6. NELs for Disturbances of the Respiratory System

SUBSTANCE, REPORT YEAR	NEL	EFFECT THAT NEL PROTECTS AGAINST	SWEDISH OEL	OEL/NEL
Aluminum (1982)	0.1–2.7 mg/m^3	Pulmonary fibrosis (occurred at 1–10 mg/m^3 but not at 0.1–2.7 mg/m^3 respirable dust)	4 mg/m^3	⩾1.5
Cobalt (1983)	0.03 mg/m^3	Asthma (induction at 0.05–0.10 mg/m^3; below 0.03 mg/m^3 only reversible effects reported)	0.05 mg/m^3	1.7
Piperazine (1985)	0.3 mg/m^3	Asthma	0.3 mg/m^3	1.0

effects than irritation of eyes and mucous membranes, and on average, lower OEL/NEL ratios would be expected for the more serious effects.

The 12 substances for which an EL could be inferred are listed in Table 4.7. Ten of them have OELs. Only two of these have an OEL/EL ratio below 1.0, and the geometric mean of the ten OEL/EL ratios is 1.8–1.9. For four of the ten substances, the EL refers to an irreversible effect. The geometric mean of the OEL/EL ratios for these four substances is 2.0.

These ratios are much higher than the OEL/EL ratios for irritation of eyes and upper passages that were reported in Table 4.5 (geometric mean, 0.47–0.58). Again, this finding runs counter to what would be expected from the relative severity of the two types of health effects.

The mean ratios reported for respiratory and irritative effects can be summarized as follows:

OEL/EL, respiratory disease	1.8–1.9
OEL/NEL, respiratory disease	⩾1.4
OEL/EL, irritation	0.47–0.58
OEL/NEL, OEL/TL, irritation	0.42–0.47

TABLE 4–7. ELs for Disturbances of the Respiratory System

SUBSTANCE, REPORT YEAR	EL	EFFECT AT EL	SWEDISH OEL	OEL/EL
Vanadium (1983)	0.06 mg/m³	Bronchial irritation and coughing (reversible)	0.2 mg/m³	3.3
Sulfur dioxide (1985)	1 ppm	Increased pulmonary resistance in volunteers (reversible)	2 ppm	2.0
Coal dust (1986)	2 mg/m³	An estimated 1% risk of developing coalworkers' pneumoconiosis (CWP) and a 0.3% risk of developing progressive massive fibrosis (PMF) (irreversible)	3 mg/m³	1.5
Nitrogen dioxide (1986)	0.5 mg/m³	Increased pulmonary resistance (reversible)	4 mg/m³	8.0
Cotton dust (1986)	0.3–0.5 mg/m³	Reduced lung function (reversible)	0.5 mg/m³	1.0–1.7
Terpenes (1987)	125 mg/m³	Bronchial irritation, reduced lung function (irreversible)	150 mg/m³	1.2
Ozone (1987)	0.24 mg/m³	Lower scores on some lung function tests after heavy exercise (reversible)	0.2 mg/m³	0.83
Diisocyanates and poly-isocyanates (1988)	1 ppb	Reduced lung function (irreversible)	5 ppb	5.0

TABLE 4-7 Continued

SUBSTANCE, REPORT YEAR	EL	EFFECT AT EL	SWEDISH OEL	OEL/EL
Titanium dioxide (1989)	0.2–2.8 mg/m^3	Reduced ventilation capacity and thickened pleura (irreversible)	5 mg/m^3	>1.8
Paper dust (1990)	<5 mg/m^3	Irritation of upper and lower passages (reversible)	2 mg/m^3	≥0.4
Attapulgite (1991)	2.7 mg/m^3	Pneumoconiosis (irreversible)	—	—
Talc, asbestos-free and with low quartz content (1992)	1 mg/m^3	Declining lung function at exposure levels below 1 mg/m^3 (irreversible)	—	—

Hence, the order of the ratios is much less reasonable than the opposite order would have been. (Note that high ratios represent a low degree of protection.)

EFFECTS ON THE NERVOUS SYSTEM

For nine substances, the critical effect was a disturbance of the central nervous system (CNS). For one of them (halothane) a NEL can be found in the consensus report, and for five others ELs can be found. For three substances no dose–effect relationship in humans was reported.[9]

For halothane, the committee reported that a prolonged complex reaction time has been observed at 17,600 mg/m^3 but not at 1760 mg/m^3. Based on this finding, a NEL of 1760 mg/m^3 can be deduced. Since the OEL is 40 mg/m^3, this yields an OEL/NEL ratio of 0.02.

TABLE 4–8. ELs for CNS Disturbances

SUBSTANCE, REPORT YEAR	EL	EFFECT AT EL	SWEDISH OEL	OEL/EL
Methyl chloroform (1981)	500 ppm	Headache, dizziness, fatigue	50 ppm	0.1
Methyl bromide (1988)	35 ppm	Slight subjective neurological symptoms	5 ppm	0.14
Methyl chloride (1992)	35 ppm	Worsened performance on vigilance and coordination tests (subjects exposed for ≥2 years)	50 ppm	1.4
Styrene (1989)	<25 mg/m^3	Higher than normal frequencies of neuropsychiatric symptoms	90 mg/m^3	≥3.6
Manganese, inorganic (1991)	0.2 mg/m^3	Early symptoms of Parkinson's disease, including prolonged reaction time and poorer performance on psychometric tests	1 mg/m^3	5.0

The five substances with ELs are summarized in Table 4.8. The geometric mean of their OEL/EL ratios is 0.81. The most striking feature of this table is the strange relation between OEL/EL ratios and the severity of the effect recorded at the EL. Manganese, which gives rise to early symptoms of Parkinson's disease at the EL, could be expected to have the lowest OEL/EL ratio among these substances. Methyl chloroform, which only produces headaches, dizziness, and fatigue at the EL, could be expected to have the highest OEL/EL ratio. To the contrary, however, manganese has the highest OEL/EL ratio in the table (5.0) and methyl chloroform the lowest (0.1). No explanation of this surprising finding has been found.

For three substances (n-hexane, methyl ethyl ketone, and 2-hexanone), the critical effect was a disturbance of the peripheral nervous system (PNS), in all three cases polyneuropathy. Dose-related information based on experience in humans was given only for one of these substances, n-hexane. The lowest concentration of n-hexane reported to cause polyneuropathy was 40–90 ppm. Since the OEL is 25 ppm, this corresponds to an OEL/EL ratio of 0.28–0.63.

OTHER NONMALIGNANT CRITICAL EFFECTS

Eight substances had critical effects on the *blood and blood-forming organs*.[10] Only for one of them, nitrogen monoxide, did the consensus report contain dose–effect information on humans, so that an EL could be inferred. The critical effect for this substance was an increased methemoglobin level, which could be observed after 15 minutes of exposure to 18 mg/m^3. Since the OEL is 30 mg/m^3, the OEL/EL ratio is 1.7.

For four of the six substances that had critical effects on the *liver* dose–effect information was lacking,[11] and a fifth has no Swedish OEL.[12] For the remaining substance, allyl chloride, the committee reports: ''Liver damage has been diagnosed in persons exposed to allyl chloride in the range 1 to 113 ppm for 16 months, and seen in experimental animals exposed to 8 ppm for 5 weeks.'' Since the OEL is 1 ppm, this yields an OEL/EL ratio of 0.01–1.

Two substances, 1,3,5-trichlorobenzene and cadmium, had disorders of the *kidney* as critical effects. No dose–effect information was available for 1,3,5-trichlorobenzene. The committee reported three times on cadmium (1981, 1984, and 1992). In the last report it concluded: "It has been estimated that it takes 25 years of occupational exposure to a cadmium concentration of 10 to 20 µg/m³ in order to reach a cadmium concentration of 200 mg/kg in renal cortex, and that approximately 10% of those with this concentration begin to develop tubular dysfunction." Taking 10–20 µg/m³ for the EL, since the OEL is 50 µg/m³ we have an OEL/EL ratio of 2.5–5.0.

Two substances, dinitrotoluene and Freon 22, had critical effects on the *heart*. Dose-related information was available only for the latter. The lowest level at which Freon 22 was reported to affect the heart (increased palpitations) was 300 ppm. Since the OEL is 500 ppm, the OEL/EL ratio is 1.7.

For two substances, triethyl amine and dimethylethylamine, the critical effect was disturbances of the *eye* (other than mere irritation), in both cases including corneal edema.

For triethyl amine, 5 mg/m³ was reported to result in "[n]o eye trouble" and 10–15 mg/m³ in swelling of the cornea after 1 to 4 hours of occupational exposure. Since the OEL is 8 mg/m³, the OEL/NEL ratio is 1.6.

For dimethylethylamine, the committee reported that experimental exposure "has caused eye irritation, visual problems and corneal edema in persons exposed to 40 mg/m³ for 8 hours. These symptoms did not appear after exposure to 20 mg/m³. . . . There are no data on long-term exposure." Since the OEL is 6 mg/m³, the OEL/NEL ratio is 0.3.[13]

For two substances, indium and ethyl glycol, the critical effect was *fetotoxicity or teratogenicity*. No dose-related information based on human exposure was available for either of these substances. However, in its report on ethyl glycol in 1982, the committee made an unusual statement about the relevance of animal experiments:

> For ethyl glycol, the critical effects seem to be those on the fetus, and functional disturbances have been documented at the present Swedish occupational exposure limit (100 ppm). Physical abnormalities have been

observed at somewhat higher air concentrations (160 ppm). There is no evidence that humans should be less sensitive to teratogenic effects than the experimental animals used. Exposures at presently allowed levels thus carry a clear risk for teratogenic effects.

When this was written, the Swedish OEL was 100 ppm. It has since then been reduced to 5 ppm, which means a reduction of the OEL/EL ratio from 1.0 to 0.05.

For selenium compounds, a consensus report in 1985 stated that a *metallic taste* was the critical effect, but in a later report on the same group of substances (1993), this statement was (implicitly) retracted, and the committee now said that no critical effect could be determined for selenium compounds. The committee's former chairman, Bo Holmberg, has informed me that in 1993 the committee considered the neurological effects of selenium to be probably more serious than the metallic taste, but due to lack of dose-related information it was unable to identify a critical effect.

For one substance, silver, *discoloration of tissues* (argyria) was given as the critical effect. It was said to appear at 0.25 mg/m^3 but not at 0.01 mg/m^3. The OEL is 0.1 mg/m^3 for the metal and 0.01 mg/m^3 for soluble compounds. Hence, the OEL/NEL ratio is 10 for the former and 1.0 for the latter. (Argyria can result from exposure either to the metal or to its compounds.)

One substance, zinc, had *metal fume fever* as its critical effect. The committee complained—as it often does—that adequate data were lacking but mentioned that there are "incompletely reported observations of metal fume fever resulting from exposure to less than 5 mg/m^3." The OEL is 5 mg/m^3, and hence the OEL/EL ratio is >1.0.

No dose–effect information was given in the consensus reports for the substances that had as critical effects *genotoxicity or mutagenicity*[14]; an effect on the *thyroid*,[15] the *reproductive system*,[16] or the *skin*[17]; or discomfort caused by *odor*.[18]

CANCER

For 15 substances, cancer was reported to be the critical effect.[19] For two of these substances, benzene and synthetic inorganic mineral fibers, critical levels or thresholds have been proposed.

The first consensus report on benzene (1981) was also the first in which the phrase "critical level" was used. In previous consensus reports, neither "critical levels" nor "critical effects" had been mentioned. The committee said that "[i]t seems reasonable to assume that the critical level for increased risk of leukemia is around 10 ppm. At any rate, there is no sure evidence of increased risk at lower levels." The OEL was 5 ppm at the time and is now 0.5 ppm. In the second report on benzene (1988), no critical level or threshold was given.

In a 1987 report on synthetic inorganic mineral fibers, the committee said that the critical effect is "the possible carcinogenic effect," primarily the increased risk of lung cancer. Furthermore, it said that "the lowest harmful level may be in the interval between 0.05 and 0.5 f/ml, though the lower limit is particularly uncertain." (The present OEL is 1 fiber/ml.)

Dose–response relationships have been indicated for six substances, with cancer as the critical effect. One of these (erionite) does not have an OEL in Sweden. For the remaining five, the following information was given:

Asbestos is a group of mineral fibers that has been extensively used in cement products (such as pipes), fire-resistant textiles, brake linings, and so on. Asbestos is banned in Sweden due to its carcinogenicity, but it still poses a health threat in repair work and in the demolition of buildings.

In a 1981 report, the committee referred to a more extensive criteria document that it had itself commissioned. That document concluded that "the lung cancer risk in three separate studies, by three different groups, is between 5 and 9% per f-yr/ml of asbestos exposure. A worker employed for 40 years in such circumstances to an exposure of 0.5 f/ml may have double the risk of death from lung cancer and an increased risk of death from 4 to 13%. Of most importance, *six* studies indicate that an asbestos exposure of 2.5 f/ml for 40 years will *at least* double the risk of lung cancer and increase total mortality by 10%" (Nicholson 1981). The current OEL is 0.2 f/ml. A simple linear extrapolation indicates that exposure at the current OEL leads to an increase in total mortality of at least 1%.

Arsenic is a metalloid and a classic poison. It is used as a pesticide and in the production of glassware, pyrotechnics, and semiconductors. Sweden is a major exporter of arsenic.

In the first of their two reports on this substance (1980), the Criteria Group performed a "mental exercise": If 1000 persons more than 65 years of age have been exposed to 10 µg/m^3 for more than 25 years, then 0.7 additional deaths in lung cancer per year can be expected. If they have been exposed to 50 µg/m^3, then 3.5 extra deaths per year can be expected. The current OEL is 30 µg/m^3, and a simple intrapolation indicates that 2.1 extra deaths due to lung cancer per year can be expected among 1000 exposed persons. In the second report on arsenic (1984), two other estimates were referred to, and the estimate in the previous report was said to be "about midway" between the two.

Ethylene oxide is a gas that is used to sterilize medical equipment and to fumigate foods and spices. It is also an intermediate in chemical synthesis.

The committee noted in 1981 that chromosome damages "which indicate cytogenetic effects, have been noted in workers who, at least for the two years prior to the study, were probably exposed to levels no higher than about 2 mg/m^3." The present OEL is 2 mg/m^3, and hence the OEL/EL ratio for cytogenetic effects is 1.0.

Chromium is a metal that is used in many alloys, including stainless steel. Welding of such materials causes exposure to chromium.

The committee said in 1993 that "[t]he highest documented risk in an epidemiological study is presented in a cohort exposed to zinc chromate. There were six cases of lung cancer in a group of 24 highly exposed (0.5–1.5 mg/m^3) men, which yields an absolute risk of 15 cases of lung cancer per 1,000 man years. This corresponds to a 'unit risk' of 1.3×10^{-1} (or 1 case per 100,000 persons per µg Cr^{VI}/m^3). This is about ten times higher than the figures calculated for Cr^{VI} compounds by the EPA . . .." The present OEL for chromates is 20 µg Cr/m^3, which then corresponds to 20 cases per 100,000 persons.

Benzene is a colorless liquid that was once a major solvent. Due to its carcinogenicity, it has now been replaced by other solvents. However, since benzene is present in crude oil, workers in petroleum-based industries are still exposed to it.

Reporting on this substance (1988), the committee quoted two studies according to which 40 ppm × year causes about 10 extra leukemia cases per 1000 workers. The present OEL is 0.5 ppm. According to a simple (but possibly misleading) linear extrapolation, among workers exposed to the OEL for their whole working-lives, an excess leukemia incidence of five cases per 1000 workers can be expected.

Unfortunately, the committee has chosen different and not directly comparable ways of presenting its risk estimates for different carcinogens. Its chairman, Johan Högberg, has informed me that the committee refrains from extrapolations (linear or otherwise) to lower doses, since it considers this to be a policy issue that is more appropriately dealt with by the Regulations Group.

THE QUALITY OF NO-EFFECT LEVELS

In most cases, the quality of NELs (or TLs) cannot be judged from the consensus reports alone. A careful study of the scientific sources is also needed.

A simple method was available for selecting a sample of NELs for detailed study. Only in five of the consensus reports was a NEL specified in the short Conclusions section that summarizes the report. These five cases were selected for scrutiny.

For one of the five substances, the committee has retracted the NEL.

In the Conclusion of its report in 1985 on selenium compounds, it claimed that "[s]elenium oxides at air concentrations below 0.1 ppm Se have not been associated with toxic effects, and here as well the metallic taste seems to be the critical effect." This statement cannot be found (either in the Conclusion or elsewhere) in their second report (1993) on selenium compounds. For the remaining four substances, the no-effect statement in the Conclusion remains unretracted.

Cobalt is a metal that is used in steel alloys.
Summarizing its report on cobolt (1982), the committee said that "the critical effects are probably those on the respiratory passages. For concentrations below 0.03 mg Co/m^3, the effects seem to be reversible, but the data indicate that chronic effects can occur at exposures between 0.05 and 0.1 mg Co/m^3 (and above)." The only ground for this statement that could be found in the report was a reference to an American report (Lichtenstein et al. 1975) on medical examinations of 22 tungsten carbide grinders, all of whom had shift time-weighted average exposures above 0.03 mg/m^3. This article contains no information on the health status of workers exposed to cobalt at concentrations below 0.03 mg/m^3.

Dimothylformamide is a colorless liquid that is used as a solvent and as a raw material in the production of synthetic fibers.
In the summary of its report on dimethylformamide (1983), the committee said: "Disturbance of alcohol metabolism, gastritis-like symptoms and liver damage seem to be the critical effects. Studies of occupational exposure indicate that air concentrations below 30 mg/m^3 (10 ppm) produce neither observable toxic effects nor antabus-like reactions." In spite of the plural "studies," only one study was cited to substantiate this conclusion: a Belgian study of 22 workers exposed to the substance in an acrylic fiber factory (Lauwerys et al. 1980). According to the cited article, liver function tests were made, but no interviews, questionnaires, or medical examinations are reported. The authors concluded that "exposure to DMF vapor for 5 years at a level usually below 30 mg/m^3 does not seem to entail a risk of liver cytolysis. It should be stressed, however, that in this factory, the selection criteria at the

beginning of employment are rather severe. Nevertheless, despite the apparently 'safe' exposure conditions, some workers reported experiencing signs of alcohol intolerance (antabuse effect) at the end of the day when they had been exposed to peak concentrations of DMF vapor (e.g., during spinneret cleaning). This indicates that interference with alcohol metabolism still occurs at an exposure below that causing liver cytolysis." In the abstract, the authors emphasized that even 10 mg/m^3 (3 ppm) "does not necessarily preclude episodes of alcohol intolerance in some workers." Hence, this article does not corroborate the statement in support of which it was cited by the Criteria Group, namely, that 30 mg/m^3 (10 ppm) produces neither observable toxic effects nor antabus-like reactions.

Piperazine is a white, crystalline substance that is used as a raw material in the manufacture of medicines, insecticides, fibers, textile dyes, and various other products.

Summarizing its report on piperazine (1984), the committee said: "The critical effect . . . seems to be induction of asthma. . . . In one factory, several cases of asthma were precipitated by a time-weighted average of 1.2 mg/m^3, though there were brief exposure peaks of 100 mg/m^3 or higher. There were no new cases noted in a workplace where the average concentration was 0.3 mg/m^3. It is not clear, however, whether it is the total dose or the brief high exposures that are critical to asthma induction." This information was based on a Swedish study of employees in a factory in which piperazine was handled (Hagmar et al. 1982). No new cases of asthma had been found in one part of the factory, where the average concentration of piperazine was 0.3 mg/m^3. (However, attacks were provoked in previously sensitized workers.) The absence of new asthma cases was concluded from (1) the absence of such case records from the company health service and (2) inquiries among present employees. No details were given about these inquiries. The number of workers in this part of the factory was not reported, nor was their length of employment. No medical or physiological examinations of the workers exposed to 0.3 mg/m^3 seem to have been performed.

Dipropylene glycol monomethyl ether is a colorless liquid that is used as a solvent and as a constituent of cosmetic products.

In the Conclusion to its report on this substance (1990), the committee said: "The critical effect... is irritation of mucous membranes. The limit for irritation has been reported to be 450 mg/m^3 (74 ppm)." The reference on which this is based is a table published by J. H. Ruth (1986) that contains odor thresholds and "irritating conc[entrations]" for various substances. In that table, the "irritating conc[entration]" of dipropylene glycol monomethyl ether is said to be 450 mg/m^3. However, the source of this value is not given. (A list of 24 sources is given, from which the table has been compiled.) Furthermore, the notion of an "irritating concentration" is not defined. Some of the other irritating concentrations given in Ruth's table are not the lowest levels at which irritation occurs. Four examples should be sufficient to show this: (1) The irritating concentration of ammonia is said to be 72 mg/m^3. As Table 4.5 shows, irritation caused by ammonia has been noticed at 35 mg/m^3. (2) The irritating concentration of 1,4-dioxane is said to be 792 mg/m^3 (= 220 ppm). As Table 4.5 shows, irritation caused by 1,4-dioxane has been noticed at 50 ppm. (3) The irritating concentration of formaldehyde is said to be 1.5 mg/m^3 (= 1.22 ppm). As Table 4.5 shows, irritation caused by formaldehyde has been noticed at 0.05 ppm. (4) The irritating concentration of phthalic anhydride is said to be 30 mg/m^3. As Table 4.5 shows, irritation caused by phthalic anhydride has been noticed at 0.2 mg/m^3. It must be concluded that Ruth's table does not provide us with thresholds, but simply with "irritating conc[entrations,]" as Ruth himself calls them. Hence, the Criteria Group's contention that 450 mg/m^3 has been put forward as a "limit for irritation" is not substantiated by the reference given in support of it.

The scientific support of these four NELs is not impressive. Each of them is based on only one article in the occupational health literature. In one case (dimethylformamide), the article warned against adverse effects at the level it was claimed to corroborate as a NEL. In another case (cobalt), the article contained no information on the health status of workers exposed to the alleged NEL. In the third case (dipropylene glycol monomethyl ether), the source turned out to be a table with no references to the origin of its values, and a value from a column containing ELs was used by the committee as a TL. Only in the fourth case (piperazine) did the article contain information about a group of workers who did not experience the critical effect of the substance after exposure to the level referred to. However, in this case, basic information such as the number of workers and the duration of exposures was missing from the article.

CONCLUSIONS

Like the German MAKs, the Swedish OELs are based on comprehensive and generally reliable summaries of the toxicological literature. They are also regularly updated—not yearly but on average every three years. The division in Sweden of the standard-setting process into two distinct parts, one scientific and one regulative, is clearly an improvement over the procedures employed by most other standard-setting bodies. Furthermore, the Swedish exposure limits are on average lower and thus more protective than those of other countries.

Nevertheless, the regulatory ratios (OEL/EL, OEL/NEL, and OEL/TL) for many substances are too high for the exposure limit to protect against the critical effect. Another disturbing finding is that these ratios are on average higher for some types of serious effects, such as respiratory diseases and CNS effects, than for less serious effects such as irritation of eyes and mucous membranes. In addition, the important distinction between ELs and NELs appears to be lost in the decision-making process. Hence, in spite of the positive achievements of the Swedish OEL system, much remains to be done to develop fully satisfactory procedures for standard setting and to provide workers with standards that protect them adequately against hazardous substances.

5

SETTING BETTER STANDARDS

In this final chapter, I will offer some proposals for the development of better standards to protect workers against potentially toxic substances. Any such proposals must be based, at least in part, on values and decision principles that go beyond the limits of science. Policy recommendations cannot be derived from science, but they should be compatible with science.

AN IMPOSSIBLE TASK?

To set OELs is no easy task. It can even be argued that the task is impossible due to conflicting demands and incomplete data.

Workers exposed to potentially dangerous substances expect exposure limits and other regulations to protect their health: Exposures at or below the limit should not give rise to disease. The other major demand on OELs, primarily represented by employers, is that the costs of compliance should be kept as low as possible: OELs should impose only such costs as are necessary to protect the health of employees.

Unfortunately, full protection of health is not easily achieved. Due to the uncertainties inherent in toxicology and epidemiology, there are virtually no safe nonzero levels of toxic exposure. That this is so for many (or all) genotoxic carcinogens is generally recognized. For these substances, the risk is not known to be eliminated until the exposure has been eliminated. Once epistemic uncertainty is taken into account, it is clear that the same is true for other substances as well. To choose limits below which no harmful effects are known to occur is no guarantee of safety. Experience shows that more often than not, such levels have to be adjusted downwards when more information becomes available.

Basically, the only way to protect against unknown health effects is to apply large safety margins (uncertainty factors). This policy can be based on the reasonable assumption that many unknown dangers lurk between the levels with known dangers and the lower levels to which the safety factors take us. But although such dangers are present for many substances, for many others they are not. Hence, protection of health can be achieved only at the price of costly measures, many of which are unnecessary in the sense that they would not be needed if we had access to perfect toxicological information.

Is the setting of OELs an impossible task? The answer depends on what is required of the OELs. It is impossible to set OELs that fully satisfy the two demands of protecting health and avoiding unnecessary costs. But if the demands are tempered, the task may not be impossible after all. The first step in solving the problem is to reformulate it: The task is not to satisfy the two demands fully, but to find a reasonable compromise between them.

To find such a compromise is a science-based enterprise in the sense of using scientific information but not in the sense of being based exclusively on science. It is in fact both science based and value based.

HEALTH-BASED EXPOSURE LIMITS

How can a defensible compromise be reached between the protection of health and counteracting factors such as economic, technological, or political feasibility? An analogy with clinical medicine can be helpful in the search for an answer.

Clinical medicine is not based on science alone. It also involves practices that have a strong ethical component. When choosing the treatments to be offered to patients, the medical community takes into account the positive and negative effects of various alternatives, weighing risks against benefits. Although these decisions are difficult and often vital, they are seldom questioned outside of the medical community. Clinical medicine is value laden, but the values it incorporates are in general uncontroversial.

One important reason for this is that medical practices are potentially *self-inflicting*. The treatments that doctors recommend to their patients are those that they would choose for themselves. We can therefore think of physicians as (more knowledgeable) representatives of their patients. This is crucial for the legitimacy of clinical medicine. Our trust in the medical system would not be the same if there were special treatments offered only to doctors and their families.

Many regulatory decisions on social risks are self-inflicting in the same sense. The persons—whether scientists, administrators, judges, or politicians—who decide on the exposure limits for atmospheric pollutants themselves breathe the air they regulate. Similarly, those who regulate food and drinking water eat the food and drink the water they regulate. The compromise between health and economics that they settle for—for it is certainly a compromise in this case as well—is imposed not only on others but also on themselves.

In contrast, decisions on OELs are nowhere self-inflicting. In fact, they cannot be so due to the division of labor in society. Only in Utopia do decision makers work in chemical factories in the morning and in administrative offices in the afternoon.

Even if OELs cannot be self-inflicting, they can at least in principle be *adjusted to the same level of risk taking as that of self-inflicting standards*. In other words, they can be based on the same criteria of acceptability as those used for food additives or drinking water. Since such self-inflicting standards reflect more general opinions in society of what is medically acceptable, in what follows they will be called *medical values*. The word *medical* does not refer here to medical science alone but to the complex and value-laden practice of clinical medicine.

Such medical values will in many cases be drastically lower than current OELs. Therefore, they probably cannot be adopted in the near future as general-purpose exposure limits. It is more realistic to think of them as starting points from the health side of what must in the end be a compromise between health and economics.

LEVELS OF AGGREGATION

The compromise between health and economics can take place on at least four different levels of aggregation. On the *workplace level*, decisions apply to particular workplaces. One company may be allowed to expose its workers, say, to 20 ppm of styrene since it cannot afford to do better, whereas another company that uses styrene in the same process is required to reduce exposures to 5 ppm.

Next comes the *work process level*. A regulation on this level applies to all companies that use a substance in the same type of work process. Thus all companies that use toluene as a component in paints are subject to the same exposure limit, whereas companies that use it as a source chemical in synthesis may be subject to another exposure limit.

The third level is the *substance level*. A regulation on this level applies to all companies that use a particular substance, irrespective of the work process. Each substance has the same exposure limit on all workplaces.

The fourth and final level is the *chemicals level*. If the compromise between health and economics is made on this level, then the level of accepted risk is the same for all substances in all workplaces.

Since the German MAKs are declared to be purely health-based, they should in principle represent a compromise on the chemicals level. As we saw in Chapter 3, this is not actually the case. In practice, the German MAKs, like all other OELs, represent a compromise on the third level, the substance level.

The basic choice of a regulatory strategy for occupational exposures has been very little discussed. I have seen no sign in the literature of any awareness that OELs, as presently constructed, represent a compromise on one of several possible levels, and that an argument is needed to show that this is the best level—if indeed it is.[1]

Considerations of cost effectiveness speak strongly for the choice of the lowest possible level of aggregation. To see this, let us first consider the chemicals level, according to which the standard of acceptability should be the same for all substances in all workplaces. Suppose that in the production of plastic boats a particular substance, such as styrene, is very expensive to eliminate. A high OEL, say 20 ppm, is admitted for styrene in order not to put an important branch of industry out of business. Furthermore, suppose that another substance, toluene, is about as dangerous at 100 ppm as styrene is at 20 ppm. Exposure to toluene can, however, be reduced inexpensively to much lower levels in all workplaces where it is used. It is, in other words, highly cost effective to reduce exposures to toluene. Then why should they not be reduced? Or, in more humanitarian terms: *How can the fact that some workers have to be exposed to high levels of one substance justify exposure of other workers to high levels of another substance?*

This argument can be brought down to the substance level. An interesting example is the exposure limit for benzene (1 ppm) that was adopted by OSHA in 1987. Values lower than this were considered infeasible due to the high cost of compliance in the petrochemicals, coke, and coal chemicals industries. These industries contained only 2.2% of the American workers exposed to benzene (Rappaport 1993, p. 686). The remaining 97.8% of the workers exposed to benzene (about 230,000 individuals) received weak protection against occupational cancer because they had the bad lack of being exposed to a substance that is also used in other work environments where it is more difficult to eliminate.[2] *How can the fact that some workers have to be exposed to high levels of a substance justify exposure of workers using the substance in a different work process to equally high levels?*

We can, of course, continue in the same way on the work process level. *How can the fact that some workers have to be exposed to high levels of a substance justify exposure of workers using the same substance in the same work process in a different workplace to equally high levels?*

All of this argues for regulating at the lowest possible level of aggregation, namely, the workplace level. There are, however, two major counterarguments against the workplace level. One is the *administrative workload*. It would be forbiddingly resource-consuming to determine exposure limits for each workplace. The other is *fairness of competition*. Any two companies undertaking the same work process should be subject to the same regulations.

The work process level fares much better with respect to these counterarguments. The argument of fair competition has virtually no bearing on that level. Companies that use the same substance in different processes are not typically in direct competition. With regard to the administrative workload, it must be conceded that regulation on the work process level is more resource-consuming than the present practice of regulating on the substance level. However, since most other occupational health and safety regulations refer to particular work processes, this cannot be an insurmountable obstacle. The work process level is the lowest feasible level of aggregation, and this is a strong reason for choosing it. *Compromises between health and economics should not be made on the substance level (the same for all uses of a substance) but on the work process level (different for different uses of a substance).*

One way to implement different exposure limits for different work processes is to provide for each substance (*1*) a *default* value to be applied if no specific exception has been made and (*2*) a list of work processes for which specified, higher *exception values* are applicable. Preferably, the default values should (after a transitional period) be medical values in the sense defined above. This is, of course, a way of adjusting the standards of proof to provide greater protection for the worker: Unless sufficient reasons for an exception have been put forward, the low default values will be applied.

Due to the rapid development of technology, assessments of economic and technological feasibility will often be outdated within a few years. Therefore, exception values should have limited validity and be revised on a regular basis. It should also be possible for the regulating body to announce changes in exposure limits several years in advance, giving companies a reasonable time to adjust to stricter demands.

The major advantage of this system is that compromises are restricted to those work processes for which they are needed. Another advantage is that the misrepresentation of OELs as ''safe values'' loses whatever credibility it may have.

A RESIDUAL EXPOSURE LIMIT

In most industrialized countries, food additives are regulated by means of a *positive list* of permitted additives for which maximal concentrations are given. Substances not included in the list are not allowed; in other words, what is not covered by the regulation is forbidden. The same principle applies to the regulation of pesticides and of medical drugs. Lists of OELs differ from these in being *negative lists*. What is not covered by a specific item on the list is allowed as far as the list is concerned. (It may, of course be prohibited under some other regulation [Zielhuis and Wibowo 1989, p. 579].)

For obvious reasons, a positive list offers better protection against adverse health effects. Unfortunately, a direct transition from the negative to the positive approach is not practical in occupational standard setting. This would require the prohibition of all substances used in workplaces that have not been assigned an exposure limit, and there are tens of thousands of such substances. However, an important step in that direction can be taken by introducing a *residual value*, a limit for the total exposure to substances that have no specific exposure limit. The list of OELs would then contain a clause such as the following:

The total exposure to substances not included in this list may not exceed x mg/m^3.

Several lists of OELs do contain a general limit for dusts (3 or 5 mg/m^3).[3] However, this limit is intended for "nonhazardous" substances. A residual value should be much lower, and it should cover vapors and mists in addition to dusts.[4] Probably the most practicable approach is to first introduce an unsatisfactorily high but enforceable residual OEL (such as 1 mg/m^3), which is then gradually reduced.

With the introduction of a residual OEL, responsibility for the documentation of new OELs can be transferred from government agencies to industry, by analogy with the already existing system for pesticides. If a company wishes to bring a new pesticide to market, it has (at least in most industrialized countries) to submit the required toxicological documentation. Similarly, a company that wishes an OEL higher than the residual value to be introduced for a new substance should be responsible for providing the necessary documentation.

INTERPRETATIVE CONSERVATIVITY

The use of toxicological, epidemiological, and other scientific information in setting OELs requires that data with only an indirect bearing on occupational health be interpreted for decision-making purposes. Extrapolations have to be made from effects on animals to effects on humans, from oral exposure to inhalation, and from higher to lower doses.

As we saw in Chapter 1, the standards of proof employed for deciding on scientific hypotheses are not suitable for administrative decision making. In science, the hypothesis that a substance has a harmful effect should be accepted only when fairly strict standards of evidence have been met. Decision makers with a responsibility for public health sometimes have to act against possible dangers even when the evidence is insufficient according to scientific standards. The following principle of *interpretative conservativity* can be used as the basis for toxicity assessments with a regulatory purpose:

> In the choice between diverging but scientifically sound interpretations of toxicological data, precedence should be given to those interpretations that support the most pessimistic predictions with respect to human health. (Hansson 1997a, p. 227)

One way to achieve conservativity is to establish a set of presumptions for biological interpretations, i.e., conservative principles that should be applied unless there are sufficient reasons to do otherwise. Perhaps the most well-known example is the presumption that animal carcinogens are human carcinogens.

It is essential to recognize that toxicological presumptions like this one are not intended as categorical rules. In some cases, carcinogenicity in animals is irrelevant to human health. Then the presumption has been overruled and should not be applied.

Toxicological presumptions can be seen as rules for apportioning the burden of proof. Just as in court, having the burden of proof does not mean that you cannot prove your case. It only means that if you cannot, then you lose.

Several government agencies, such as the Environmental Protection Agency (EPA) in the United States, have adopted conservative biological presumptions for the interpretation of toxicity data (Finkel 1994; NRC 1994). However, no list of OELs is based on a systematic use of such presumptions.

This is not the place to discuss the many technical issues that need to be settled in order to implement the principle of interpretative conservativity. It will suffice to show by an example how it can be put into practice.

The most common toxicological experiment involves the oral administration of a substance to a rodent. Since it takes much less to kill a mouse than to kill a human, the doses obtained in these experiments cannot be applied directly to humans. It is necessary to extrapolate the oral doses from rodents to the bigger human body.

The traditional way of doing this is to assume that toxicity is proportionate to body weight. Oral doses are expressed as weight unit per weight unit, e.g., milligrams per kilogram. Suppose, for instance, that 1 mg is the lowest dose of a substance that causes symptoms of disease in mice weighing 25 g. This dose can be expressed as 40 mg/kg. Translating this dose to humans, the same toxic effect can be expected in a person weighing 75 kg after ingesting 40 × 75 = 3000 mg of the substance.

However, it is far from self-evident that this is the right way to perform the extrapolation. Toxicity may not be proportionate to body weight. A strong argument can be made that, in general, toxicity is proportionate to the surface area of the body: Toxicity can be assumed to be (roughly speaking) proportionate to the metabolic rate. Metabolic rates are roughly proportionate to heat loss. The heat loss from warm-blooded animals is roughly proportionate to the surface areas of their bodies. Therefore, toxicity should be roughly proportionate to body surface areas.[5] (Pinkel 1958).

Let us again consider our example with the mouse weighing 25 g. Its body surface area is about 0.01 m^2. The toxic dose, 1 mg, can therefore be expressed as 100 mg/m^2.[6] The body surface area of a human weighing 75 kg is about 2.0 m^2. Therefore, the corresponding dose in humans is 100 × 2.0 = 200 mg. This is much less than the 3000 mg obtained with body weight scaling. Hence, the choice of scaling factors may be a decisive factor in administrative decisions such as the determination of OELs.

The evidence on interspecific scaling factors is inconclusive, and no consensus on the choice of an appropriate scaling method seems to be in sight among toxicologists.[7] According to the principle of interpretative conservativity, the most pessimistic of the reasonable scaling factors should be employed. This means that a toxicological presumption in favor of body-area scaling should be established. Consequently, the traditional method of expressing toxicity in relation to body weight (milligrams per kilogram) should be avoided.

Under the assumption that toxicity is roughly proportionate to metabolic rate, scaling factors are not needed for inhalation experiments. The volume of inhaled air is proportionate to the metabolic rate. Therefore, animal exposures to a certain concentration in inhaled air should be correlated with human exposure to the same concentration. Thus 200 ppm in the air for a mouse corresponds (roughly) to 200 ppm for humans.

STATISTICAL EVALUATIONS

Biological interpretations and extrapolations are not all that is needed to evaluate toxicological and epidemiological data. Statistical assessments are equally important. Their purpose is to determine, given the observations from experiments and epidemiological studies, what the underlying frequencies of disease may be.

As we saw in Chapter 1, two central technical concepts are problematic with respect to the burden of proof: statistical significance and NOELs.

Although the criterion of statistical significance helps us to avoid type I errors (measures against a nonexisting effect), it offers no protection against type II errors (no measures against an actual effect). Therefore, the information that a certain study showed no statistically significant effect needs to be supplemented with an estimate of the size of the adverse health effects that may have gone undetected in this study. Technically, this information can be obtained by calculating the *detection level* of negative tests. The detection level of a statistical test with the critical level α^* is the smallest effect (frequency difference) that would, with at least probability $1 - \alpha^*$, lead to a significant outcome of the test. Hence, the detection level of a test with the conventional critical level 0.05 is the smallest effect that would, with a probability of at least 0.95, produce a statistically significant outcome (Hansson 1995).

The conventional way to summarize a negative epidemiological study in a report to decision makers is as follows:

In a study of chemical workers who had been exposed to the substance at 50 ppm, there was no significant increase ($\alpha^* = 0.05$) in the incidence of leukemia.

To indicate the amount of safety gained from this negative result, a second sentence should be added:

In a study of chemical workers who had been exposed to the substance at 50 ppm, there was no significant increase ($\alpha^* = 0.05$) in the incidence of leukemia. The detection level for an increase in the incidence of leukemia was 1.8 cases in 100 individuals.

The conventional way to report a negative outcome from an animal experiment is as follows:

In an inhalation study on rats, no significant difference in tumor frequency was discovered at 50, 100, or 200 mg/m^3.

To this, similarly, a sentence specifying the detection level should be added:

In an inhalation study on rats, no significant difference in tumor frequency was discovered at 50, 100, or 200 mg/m^3. The detection level for an increase in tumor incidence was nine cases in 100 individuals.

In the preceding chapters, we have seen many examples of how NOELs have been misused or misunderstood. The very notion of a NOEL gives the impression that the absence of an effect, in the sense of zero frequency, can be experimentally determined. In fact, all that a no-effect experiment can provide is an upper bound on the size of a possible effect.[8] It is therefore more appropriate to talk about *bounded effect levels* rather than *no-observed-effect levels*.

The bounded effect level answers the question "How big should an effect be to be implausible, given the results that we have obtained?" where "implausible" is taken in the conventional sense of a probability below 5%.[9] Bounded effect levels come in two variants: those based on an observation at the relevant dose level and those based on extrapolation to dose levels not used in the actual experiment. The former variant will be called the *observed bounded effect level* (OBEL) and is defined as follows:

> A study has been performed with a chemical exposure at dose level D. Let x be the smallest true effect that would, with a probability of at least 0.95, give rise to a larger observed effect than the one obtained in this experiment. Then the study has shown D to be an *observed bounded effect level* for x, i.e., D is the OBEL(x) that has been obtained in the experiment.

Intuitively, if $D = \text{OBEL}(x)$, then effects from dose D can reasonably be expected to be smaller than x under the conditions of the study. The OBEL values that can be obtained from common types of experiments and epidemiological studies refer to much higher incidences of disease than those normally considered acceptable for human exposure. Therefore, we have to extrapolate to lower dose levels. The choice of an appropriate extrapolation procedure should, at least ideally, depend on the nature of the adverse effect. In the absence of adequate specific information, simple linear extrapolation can be used as a default method.

The linear extrapolations obtained from OBELs will be called LEBELs. LE stands for "linearly extrapolated."[10] The definition follows: If

$$D = \text{OBEL}(x) \text{ and } 0 < D' < D$$

then

$$D' = \text{LEBEL}\left(x \times \frac{D'}{D}\right)$$

Hence, if the experimental dose of 20 ppm was an OBEL(0.02), then LEBEL(10^{-3}) = 1 ppm and LEBEL(10^{-6}) = 0.001 ppm.

Linear extrapolation is a very rough method, but it seems to be the

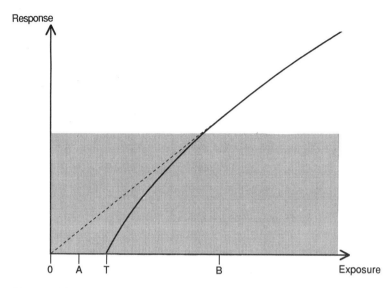

FIGURE 5.1. In the presence of a threshold for the harmful effect, linear extrapolation may lead to an overestimation of the risks at low exposure levels. The continuous line is a dose–response curve for a hypothetical substance. The gray area represents the frequencies of harmful effects that cannot be distinguished from zero in experiments of feasible size. The toxic effects of this substance do not materialize at dose levels below T, the threshold level.

An experiment is performed at dose level B. A linear extrapolation (indicated by the broken line) overestimates the true frequency of harmful effects at dose level A.

best that we can do when we have no specific information about mechanisms of toxicity. The conventional use of uncertainty factors, such as in food toxicology, depends on a similar linearity assumption. For reasons shown in Figures 5.1, 5.2, 5.3, and 5.4, linear extrapolation may either overestimate or underestimate the actual frequency of disease (Bailar et al. 1988, 1990; Park 1990; Sielken 1990; Crawford and Wilson 1996).

As an example of how LEBEL values can be used, we can take the MAK commission's report from 1993 on chloroacetic acid methyl ester

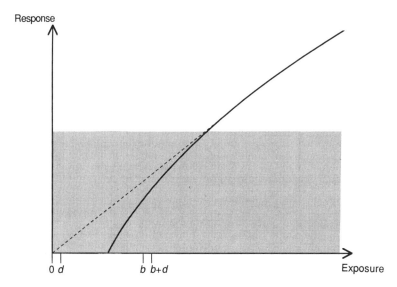

FIGURE 5.2. The presence of a threshold for the toxic effects of a substance does not necessarily mean that a small exposure to the substance is harmless. The small exposure may add to an already existing exposure to some other substance(s) with the same toxic mechanism—perhaps a naturally occurring substance that is ingested with food. In the diagram, exposure to the small dose d does not lead to an increase in total dose from 0 to d (which would be harmless) but from the background exposure b to $b + d$ (which means an enhanced toxic effect). Some researchers believe this to be a very common mechanism both for carcinogenicity and for non-carcinogenic toxicity. (Crawford and Wilson 1996)

(see the sections on "Animal No-Effect Levels" and "Standards of Evidence" in Chapter 3.) The exposure limit was set at 1 ppm as the result of applying an uncertainty factor of 10 to a NOEL of 10 ppm. This NOEL was based on a study with only ten animals. It can easily be shown that that 10 ppm = OBEL(0.26) and hence that 1 ppm = LEBEL(0.026).[11] This estimate gives a much better understanding of the statistical uncertainty inherent in the exposure limit 1 ppm than the statement that it is one-tenth of the NOEL.

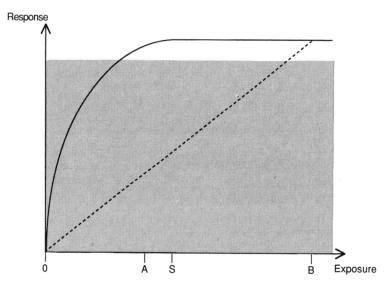

FIGURE 5.3. In the presence of a saturation mechanism, linear extrapolation may lead to an underestimation of the risks at low exposure levels. As in Figure 5.1, the gray area represents the frequencies of harmful effects that cannot be distinguished from zero in experiments of feasible size. The actual dose–response relationship for a hypothetical substance is indicated by the continuous line. The toxicity of this substance depends on bioactivation via a metabolic route that is saturated at the level marked S in the diagram. At levels higher than S, the amount of the toxic metabolite cannot be further increased.

An experiment is performed at dose level B. A linear extrapolation (indicated by the broken line) underestimates the true frequency at dose level A.

A mechanism of this type has been observed for vinyl chloride. At doses above 10,000 ppm there is no further increase in the incidence of liver angiosarcomas, which is 20–25% at that level (Bailar et al. 1988). If a similar break in the dose–response curve for some other substance occurs at 5% or at a lower incidence, then it may be virtually undetectable in normal-sized bioassays.

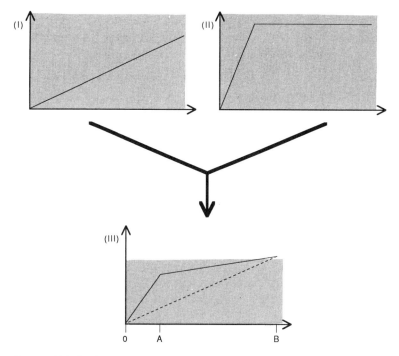

FIGURE 5.4. In the presence of a more sensitive subpopulation, linear extrapolation may lead to an underestimation of the risks at low exposure levels. Diagram I shows the dose–response relationship for a hypothetical substance in 50% of the population. Diagram II shows the corresponding relationship in the remaining 50%. The dose–response relationship for the whole population, shown in diagram III, is a weighted average of diagrams I and II. Linear extrapolation based on observations at dose level B will lead to an underestimation of the incidence of disease at dose level A. The existence of two subpopulations with different response rates may, of course, be unknown.

THE ROLE OF SCIENCE IN STANDARD SETTING

We have already concluded that any nonzero value for toxic exposure must be the outcome of a compromise between health interests and counteracting interests. Balancing various social interests against each other is not a task for which scientists are better qualified than anyone else (Hansson 1989). The organizational consequences of this can be summarized as follows:

1. *The bipartition of the regulatory task.* The decision-making process has two parts. The *scientific* part should be performed by experts in the relevant scientific fields. It derives its legitimacy from the expertise of those who perform it. The *policy* part can, in a democratic society, derive its legitimacy only from the same source as other political or administrative processes: Those who perform it represent the people, to whom they are ultimately accountable.

The Swedish organization for OEL setting is based on this bipartite structure, and the same seems to apply to its Dutch counterpart (Zielhuis and Wibowo 1989).

With this, however, the issue is not settled. The judgments that standard setters require from a scientific body cannot be defined in purely scientific terms, since the standards of evidence that are appropriate in regulatory applications may differ from those used in science. It is not sufficient to require a scientific committee to evaluate the toxicity of various substances. They must also be instructed on what standards of evidence to apply (Hansson 1993a). This leads us to the following additional organizational principle for regulatory toxicology:

2. *Policy-based interpretative practices.* Scientific evaluations for regulatory purposes should, as far as possible, be based on predetermined interpretative practices, not on ad hoc decisions made substance by substance. Policymakers must lay down basic requirements for the scientific review process, such as general standards of evidence. Scientists must transform these requirements into interpretative practices that can be used in the evaluation of individual substances.

In regulatory toxicology, all decisions are made under conditions of uncertainty. New data may show substances to have previously unknown properties, and therefore any decision may have to be revised. This unfortunate predicament is seldom explained to the public. Instead, risk assessments are often communicated in a way that creates an illusory picture of certainty (Hansson 1993b). Such misleading practices should be replaced by a policy that gives a correct picture of the epistemic situation.

3. *Recognition of uncertainty.* The scientific uncertainties inherent in OELs and other regulations should be emphasized in all communications with the public.

Scientific expert committees have a strong tendency to seek consensus and to opt for compromises whenever possible (Hansson and Johannesson 1997). The Swedish Criteria Group for OELs has gone as far as to call their reports ''consensus reports''—a clear indication that diverging opinions are not welcome. (Indeed, no minority opinion has ever been published.) It is surprising how often committees of scientists—not only in toxicology—end up with a unanimous opinion on issues that are controversial in the scientific community.

The search for consensus has many virtues, but in the regulatory context a consensus-oriented approach to science may have the effect of underplaying uncertainties. It would be much better to actively promote the publication of scientifically respectable minority opinions. Such statements are a useful way of highlighting uncertainties. Furthermore, a less consensus-oriented approach may help the majority to discover alternative interpretations of data. The following guideline is proposed:

4. *Diversity of scientific opinions.* Scientific committees that inform and advise decision makers should make no special attempt to achieve consensus. Instead, when there is a diversity of scientifically respectable opinions, they should report on this diversity.

Written minority opinions should be encouraged, and should be published along with the majority opinion.

One of the possibilities that a rational decision maker has to take into account is that the experts may be wrong—as has happened so many times in the past (Hansson 1996, 1997c).

In a regulative process that accords with these four principles, standards of acceptability are moved out of the realm of science, and so are standards of evidence (with the obvious exception of issues of technical implementation). In this way, the role of science is narrowed down to its proper field of competence. Science is a wonderful tool, but only when used for what it can accomplish. The use of science to settle value-laden policy issues is just as abusive of a wonderful tool as the use of a violin bow for a crowbar.

APPENDIX: HOW TO COMPARE EXPOSURE LIMITS

Lists of OELs record the risk assessments made by regulatory agencies. A method for comparing such lists can be used to compare these risk assessments. For obvious reasons, no conclusions about actual working conditions can be drawn from studies of exposure limits.

A comparison between two lists of exposure limits should refer to all substances that have exposure limits on both lists. For each substance, the quotient between its values on the two lists is the best indicator of the difference.[1] The key to accurate comparisons of complete lists is to compute the geometric mean of these quotients, rather than median values or arithmetic means, which were used in the few previous statistical studies of the overall development of OELs (Hansson 1982; Rappaport 1993).

An important reason for the choice of geometric means can be seen from the two hypothetical list of OELs in Table A1. The geometric mean of the three B/A quotients is 1.0, whereas the arithmetic mean is 3.7, which is unsatisfactory in view of the symmetry of the proportions.

TABLE A–1. Two Hypothetical Lists of OELs Covering the Same Substances

	LIST A	LIST B	QUOTIENT B/A
Substance 1	20 mg/m^3	200 mg/m^3	10
Substance 2	15 mg/m^3	15 mg/m^3	1
Substance 3	10 mg/m^3	1 mg/m^3	0.1

The arithmetic mean of the B/A quotients gives the incorrect impression that list B has higher values than list A, whereas the arithmetic mean of the A/B quotients, which is also 3.7, gives the opposite impression. To the contrary, for any two lists A and B, the geometric mean of A/B quotients is above 1 if and only if that of the B/A quotients is below 1. (The product of the two values is always 1.)

Geometric means of the quotients of OEL values were used in preparing Table 2.1 and Figure 2.1, which record the development of TLVs. The original TLV list from 1946 was used as a basis for comparison. This may be called the *base-year method*.

Geometric means of the quotients were also used for Table 4.1 and Figure 4.1, which show the development of Swedish OELs. In this case, however, each list of OELs was compared to its immediate predecessor. The mean quotients were multiplied to obtain the cumulative trend. Hence, the entry for 1982 in Table 4.1 was obtained by multiplying three numbers: the geometric mean of the 1975/1969 quotients, that of the 1979/1975 quotients, and that of the 1982/1979 quotients. This may be called the *adjacent-list method*.

The two methods do not differ much in their outcome for Swedish OELs. (The base-year method yields the value 0.38 for 1994 compared to the value 0.37 obtained by the adjacent-list method, which is shown in Table 4.1.) The adjacent-list method was chosen to increase the small number of substances on which comparisons for carcinogens and solvents could be based.

When several lists of OELs are compared, it is useful to have a common standard against which all of them can be measured. In other words, a standard list S should be chosen, such that the various lists

A, B, C, and so on are compared in terms of the geometric means of the quotients for A/S, B/S, C/S, and so on.

It would perhaps be natural to assume that such a standard or benchmark list has to be toxicologically reasonable—in other words, that it should contain medically sound OELs. Since our knowledge of dose–response relationships is fragmentary for many substances, such a standard would be very difficult to find. Fortunately, due to our choice of geometric means for aggregation, the relationships between different lists (i.e., the ratios between the overall values) will be the same irrespective of the values on the benchmark list. More precisely, let A and B be two lists, and let S_1 and S_2 be two candidate benchmark lists that have values for the same substances. Let $m(A,S_1)$ be the geometric mean of the A/S_1 quotients, and so on. It follows directly that:

$$\frac{m(A,S_1)}{m(B,S_1)} = \frac{m(A,S_2)}{m(B,S_2)}$$

Hence, the values assigned to substances on the benchmark list are not important. What is important, however, is the choice of substances to be included. The benchmark list should contain mainly substances that can be found on most lists of OELs. One list stands out as the one that best satisfies this criterion: the first list of TLVs from 1946 (LaNier 1984). The exposure limits on this list and its yearly successors have been the starting point for most agencies throughout the world that have issued exposure limits of their own. Therefore, most lists of OELs assign values to most of the substances on ACGIH's 1946 list.

The TLVs on the ACGIH list from 1946 came in four groups: (*1*) 110 TLVs for gases and vapors, expressed in ppm, (*2*) 19 TLVs for "toxic dusts, fumes and mists," expressed in mg/m^3, (*3*) 13 TLVs for mineral dusts, expressed in million particle per cubic foot (mppcf), and (*4*) 2 TLVs for radiations ("radon or thoron gas," respectively, "X or gamma radiation"), one of which was expressed in curies/m^3 and the other in roentgen. For most of the dusts in the third group, various units of measurement have been used on different lists of OELs, and the translation between these units (such as mg/m^3 and fibers/ml) is often uncertain. Therefore, these OELs are not included in the benchmark list. The two values in the fourth group are excluded partly for similar reasons and partly because OELs for these exposures are not normally included in modern lists of OELs.

Five values from group (*1*) have been excluded since they refer to insufficiently specified mixtures (gasoline, coal tar naphtha, petroleum naphtha, Stoddard solvent, and turpentine). The same applies to one value from group (*2*) (chlorodiphenyl). This leaves us with 105 + 18 = 123 values to be included on the benchmark list.

Some of these values refer to substances with several isomers that have not always been treated as a group in later lists of OELs. On the benchmark list, 22 substances from the ACGIH 1946 list have been further specified: *n*-amyl acetate (amyl acetate), chromic acid (chromic acid and chromates), *1,2*-dichloro-*1,1,2,2*-tetrafluoroethane (dichlorotetrafluoroethane), *N,N*-dimethylaniline (dimethylaniline), *2,4*-dinitrotoluene (dinitrotoluene), *p*-dioxane (dioxane), sodium fluoride (fluorides), *n*-heptane (heptane), *n*-hexane (hexane), iron(III)oxide (iron oxide), α-isophorone (isophorone), *3*-methyl-2-butanone (methyl butanone), *o*-methylcyclohexanone (methylcyclohexanone), *o*-nitrotoluene (nitrotoluene), nitrogen dioxide (nitrogen oxides other than nitrous oxides), *n*-pentane (pentane), 2-pentanone (pentanone), *n*-propyl acetate (propyl acetate), *2,4,6*-tetryl (tetryl), *o*-toluidine (toluidine), *2,4,6*-trinitrotoluene (trinitrotoluene), and *o*-xylene (xylene). The complete benchmark list, with these modifications included, can be found in Table A3.

The ACGIH 1946 values should be interpreted as time-weighted averages for a whole working day (TWAs). Most other lists provide ceiling values (measured during a shorter period such as 5, 10, or 30 minutes) either to replace or to supplement TWAs for some substances. When another list is compared to the benchmark list, the following procedure is applied to ceiling values:

Appendix: How to Compare Exposure Limits

TABLE A–2. A Benchmark Ceiling Value Is Obtained by Multiplying the Benchmark TWA by the "C Factor" Obtained from This Table*

TWA (PPM OR MG/M^3)	C FACTOR
$x \leq 1$	3
$1 < x \leq 10$	2
$10 < x \leq 100$	1.5
$100 < x \leq 1000$	1.25
$1000 < x$	1

*The method is adopted from the ACGIH's list of threshold limit values (see LaNier 1984).

1. If both a TWA and a ceiling value are given, then the former is compared to the benchmark TWA and the ceiling value is disregarded.
2. If only a ceiling value is given, it is compared to the benchmark ceiling value that can be obtained by multiplying the benchmark TWA with the factor recommended by the ACGIH (first in its 1963 list), as shown in Table A2.

Given a substance that appears on both an OEL list and the benchmark list, the *BL quotient* for that substance is the quotient between its value on the OEL list and its value on the benchmark list (calculated according to the rules for ceiling values given above). The geometric mean of all BL quotients for substances on a list of OELs can be used as a measure of the overall level of that list. This is how the values reported in Table 1.1 and Figure 1.1 have been calculated.[2]

TABLE A–3. The Benchmark List

SUBSTANCE	CAS REGISTRY NUMBER	TLV 1946
Acetaldehyde	75-07-0	200 ppm
Acetic acid	64-19-7	10 ppm
Acetone	67-64-1	500 ppm
Acrolein	107-02-8	0.5 ppm
Acrylonitrile	107-13-1	20 ppm
Ammonia	7664-41-7	100 ppm
n-Amyl acetate	628-63-7	200 ppm
Aniline	62-53-3	5 ppm
Arsine (arsenic hydride)	7784-42-1	1 ppm
Barium peroxide as Ba	1304-29-6	0.5 mg/m^3
Benzene	71-43-2	100 ppm
Bromine	7726-95-6	1 ppm
1,3-Butadiene	106-99-0	5000 ppm
n-Butanol (n-butyl alcohol)	71-36-3	50 ppm
n-Butyl acetate (1-butyl acetate)	123-86-4	200 ppm
Butyl cellosolve (2-butoxyethanol)	111-76-2	200 ppm
Cadmium	7440-43-9	0.1 mg/m^3
Carbon dioxide	124-38-9	5000 ppm
Carbon disulfide	75-15-0	20 ppm
Carbon monoxide	630-08-0	100 ppm
Carbon tetrachloride (tetrachloromethane)	56-23-5	50 ppm
Cellosolve (2-ethoxyethanol)	110-80-5	200 ppm
Cellosolve acetate (2-ethoxyethyl acetate)	111-15-9	100 ppm
Chlorine	7782-50-5	5 ppm
1-Chloro-1-nitropropane	600-25-9	20 ppm
2-Chloro-1,3-butadiene (β-chloroprene)	126-99-8	25 ppm
Chloroform (trichloromethane)	67-66-3	100 ppm
Chromic acid	7738-94-5	0.1 mg/m^3
Cyclohexane	110-82-7	400 ppm
Cyclohexanol	108-93-0	100 ppm
Cyclohexanone	108-94-1	100 ppm
Cyclohexene	110-83-8	400 ppm
1,1-Dichloro-1-nitroethane	594-72-9	10 ppm
1,2-Dichloro-1,1,2,2-tetrafluoroethane (Freon 114)	76-14-2	10000 ppm
o-Dichlorobenzene (1,2-dichlorobenzene)	95-50-1	75 ppm
Dichlorodifluoromethane (Freon 12)	75-71-8	10000 ppm

TABLE A-3 (Continued)

SUBSTANCE	CAS REGISTRY NUMBER	TLV 1946
1,1-Dichloroethane (ethylidene chloride, ethylidene dichloride)	75-34-3	100 ppm
1,2-Dichloroethane (1,2-ethylene dichloride)	107-06-2	100 ppm
1,2-Dichloroethylene (acetylene dichloride)	540-59-0	200 ppm
Dichloroethyl ether (bis(2-chloroethyl) ether)	111-44-4	15 ppm
Dichloromethane (methylene chloride)	75-09-2	500 ppm
Dichloromonofluoromethane (dichlorofluoromethane, Freon 21)	75-43-4	5000 ppm
N,N-Dimethylaniline	121-69-7	5 ppm
Dimethyl sulfate	77-78-1	1 ppm
2,4-Dinitrotoluene	121-14-2	1.5 mg/m^3
p-Dioxane (1,4-dioxane)	123-91-1	500 ppm
Ethyl acetate	141-78-6	400 ppm
Ethyl alcohol (ethanol)	64-17-5	1000 ppm
Ethyl benzene	100-41-4	200 ppm
Ethyl bromide (monobromoethane)	74-96-4	400 ppm
Ethyl chloride (monochloroethane)	75-00-3	5000 ppm
Ethylene chlorohydrin (2-chloroethanol)	107-07-3	10 ppm
Ethyl ether (diethyl ether)	60-29-7	400 ppm
Ethyl formate	109-94-4	200 ppm
Ethylene oxide	75-21-8	100 ppm
Ethyl silicate (tetra ethyl orthosilicate)	78-10-4	100 ppm
Fluoride, sodium-, as F	7681-49-4	2.5 mg/m^3
Formaldehyde	50-00-0	10 ppm
n-Heptane	142-82-5	500 ppm
n-Hexane	110-54-3	500 ppm
Hydrogen chloride	7647-01-0	10 ppm
Hydrogen cyanide	74-90-8	20 ppm
Hydrogen fluoride	7664-39-3	3 ppm
Hydrogen selenide	7783-07-5	0.1 ppm
Hydrogen sulfide	7783-06-4	20 ppm
Iodine	7553-56-2	0.1 mg/m^3
Iron(III)oxide, fume	1309-37-1	15 mg/m^3
Isoamyl alcohol (3-pentanol)	584-02-1	100 ppm
α-Isophorone	78-59-1	25 ppm
Isopropanol (isopropyl alcohol)	67-63-0	400 ppm

(continued)

TABLE A-3. (Continued)

SUBSTANCE	CAS REGISTRY NUMBER	TLV 1946
Isopropyl ether (diisopropyl ether)	108-20-3	500 ppm
Lead	7439-92-1	0.15 mg/m³
Magnesium oxide, fume	1309-48-4	15 mg/m³
Manganese	7439-96-5	6 mg/m³
Mercury	7439-97-6	0.1 mg/m³
Mesityl oxide (4-methyl-3-penten-2-one)	141-79-7	50 ppm
Methanol (methyl alcohol)	67-56-1	200 ppm
3-Methyl-2-butanone (methyl isopropyl ketone)	563-80-4	200 ppm
Methylcyclohexane	108-87-2	500 ppm
Methylcyclohexanol	25639-42-3	100 ppm
o-Methylcyclohexanone (2-methylcyclohexanone)	583-60-8	100 ppm
Methyl acetate	79-20-9	100 ppm
Methyl bromide (bromomethane)	74-83-9	20 ppm
Methyl cellosolve (2-methoxyethanol, ethylene glycol monomethyl ether)	109-86-4	100 ppm
Methyl cellosolve acetate (2-methoxyethyl acetate, ethylene glycol monomethyl ether acetate)	110-49-6	100 ppm
Methyl chloride (monochloromethane)	74-87-3	200 ppm
Methyl ethyl ketone (2-butanone)	78-93-3	200 ppm
Methyl formate	107-31-3	400 ppm
Methyl isobutyl ketone (4-methyl-2-pentanone)	108-10-1	200 ppm
Monochlorobenzene (chlorobenzene)	108-90-7	75 ppm
Monofluorotrichloromethane (trichloromonofluoromethane, Freon 11)	75-69-4	10000 ppm
Nitrobenzene	98-95-3	5 ppm
Nitroethane	79-24-3	200 ppm
Nitrogen dioxide	10102-44-0	25 ppm
Nitroglycerin	55-63-0	0.5 ppm
Nitromethane	75-52-5	200 ppm
o-Nitrotoluene (mononitrotoluene)	88-72-2	5 ppm
Octane	111-65-9	500 ppm
Ozone	10028-15-6	1 ppm
Pentachloronaphthalene	1321-64-8	0.5 mg/m³

TABLE A–3 (Continued)

SUBSTANCE	CAS REGISTRY NUMBER	TLV 1946
n-Pentane	109-66-0	5000 ppm
2-Pentanone (methyl propyl ketone)	107-87-9	200 ppm
Phosgene	75-44-5	1 ppm
Phosphine (hydrogen phosphide)	7803-51-2	1 ppm
Phosphorous trichloride (phosphorous chloride)	7719-12-2	0.5 ppm
n-Propyl acetate	109-60-4	200 ppm
Stibine (antimony trihydride)	7803-52-3	10 ppm
Styrene	100-42-5	400 ppm
Sulfur chloride (sulfur monochloride)	10025-67-9	1 ppm
Sulfur dioxide	7446-09-5	10 ppm
Sulfuric acid	7664-93-9	0.5 mg/m^3
Tellurium	13494-80-9	0.01 mg/m^3
1,1,2,2-Tetrachloroethane	79-34-5	10 ppm
Tetrachloroethylene (perchloroethylene)	127-18-4	200 ppm
2,4,6-Tetryl (2,4,6-trinitrophenylmethylnitramine)	479-45-8	1.5 mg/m^3
Toluene	108-88-3	200 ppm
o-Toluidine	95-53-4	5 ppm
Trichloroethylene	79-01-6	200 ppm
Trichloronaphthalene	1321-65-9	5 mg/m^3
2,4,6-Trinitrotoluene	118-96-7	1.5 mg/m^3
Vinyl chloride	75-01-4	500 ppm
o-Xylene	95-47-6	200 ppm
Zinc oxide fume	1314-13-2	15 mg/m^3

NOTES

CHAPTER 1. REGULATING THE UNKNOWN

1. The term *occupational exposure limit* (OEL) was proposed in 1977 by the International Labor Organization. It has also been accepted by the World Health Organization (Zielhuis and Wibowo 1989, p. 578). Other names for occupational exposure standards include *threshold limit value, maximum accepted concentration, maximum acceptable concentration, maximum allowed concentration, maximum allowable concentration, maximum permitted concentration*, and *permissible exposure limit*.

2. Dietl's study differed from modern clinical tests in not being randomized (Dietl 1849, p. 125).

3. One-sided reliance on statistical significance has similar effects in other fields of biomedical research. Freiman and coworkers (1978) reanalyzed "negative," i.e., nonsignificant, clinical tests and found that in most of them substantial therapeutic improvements might have gone undetected.

4. Computerized simulation studies with various experimental designs and dose–response curves have confirmed the severity of this problem (Leisenring and Ryan 1992).

5. To some extent, this effect can be compensated for by extrapolation from high-dose experiments.

CHAPTER 2. THE MOST INFLUENTIAL STANDARD

The quotation from the preamble of the TLV list is taken from: American Conference of Governmental Industrial Hygienists, Inc. (ACGIH®), *1996 Threshold Limit Values (TLVs®) for Chemical Substances and Physical Agents and Biological Exposure Indices (BEIs®)*. Reprinted with permission from the ACGIH.

The quotation from Vernon Carter's article is taken from *Annals of the American Conference of Governmental Industrial Hygienists*, 12:11–13, 1985. American Conference of Governmental Industrial Hygienists, Inc. (ACGIH®) Reprinted with permission from the ACGIH.

The quotation from Herbert Stokinger's article in the *Archives of Environmental Health* 19:277–281, 1969 is reprinted with permission of the Helen Dwight Reid Educational Foundation. Published by Heldref Publications, 1319 Eighteenth Street, NW, Washington, DC 20036-1802. Copyright © 1969.

1. In its first few years, its name was the National Conference of Governmental Industrial Hygienists (NCGIH).

2. The geometric mean has been calculated from a table provided by Robinson and coworkers (1991, pp. 6–8). They give the median (2.5) and the arithmetic mean (71.4). The choice of geometric means is explained in the Appendix. On OSHA's use of TLVs, see also articles by Paxman and Robinson (1990), Cox (1991), Vladeck and Wolfe (1991), and Sentes (1992).

3. References: Argentina (Cook 1987, p. 91), Australia (Cook 1987, pp. 91–92), Austria (Castleman and Ziem 1988, p. 531), Belgium (Lauwerys 1991), Brazil (Cook 1987, p. 93), Canada (Sentes 1989), Chile (Cook 1987, p. 94), Denmark (Cook 1987, p. 95), Germany (Woitowitz 1988, p. 225), India (Cook 1987, pp. 97–98), Indonesia (Cook 1987, p. 98), Ireland (Cook 1987, p. 98), Israel (Dror 1988; Richter 1988), Japan (Tsuchiya 1988), Malaysia (Cook 1987, p. 99), Mexico (Cook 1987, p. 99), the Netherlands (Zielhuis and Wibowo 1989, p. 579), the Philippines (Cook 1987, p. 101), Portugal (Castleman and Ziem 1988, p. 531), South Africa (Webster 1989; Myers 1991), Spain (Cook 1987, pp. 101–102), Sweden (see Chapter 4), Switzerland (Cook 1987, p. 103), Thailand (Cook 1987, p. 103), the United Kingdom (Cook 1987, pp. 103–104), Venezuela (Cook 1987, p. 106), and the former Yugoslavia (Djuric 1988).

4. Jeffrey Lee, who was later to become chairman of the ACGIH, recalled

in 1987 that after the passage of the Occupational Safety and Health Act, he believed "that TLVs would no longer be needed; that NIOSH and OSHA would under their mandates, provide the needed recommended and required occupational standards" (Lee 1987).

5. For a similar claim, see Stokinger (1984 [1981]), p. 280.

6. This applies in particular to poor Third World countries, where malnutrition and parasitic diseases are the rule rather than the exception. However, the preamble to the list of TLVs explicitly warns against the use of TLVs in "countries whose working conditions or cultures differ from those in the United States of America" (ACGIH 1996).

7. See Rappaport (1993, pp. 689–691) for some further observations on reductions in the list of TLVs.

8. See ACGIH (1990, p. 342) for corrections of some minor mistakes in Ziem and Castleman (1989), which do not alter the overall picture.

9. See Salter (1988) for a study of the workings of the TLV committee in the early 1980s.

10. Aristotle, *De Sophisticis Elenchis* 167b, 1–20.

CHAPTER 3. PURELY HEALTH-BASED VALUES?

1. Here and in what follows, references to documentation reports are made by citing the name of the substance and the year the report was adopted. These reports can all be easily found in Senatskommission (1995).

Some documentation reports have been published in official English translations (DFG 1991–1994). These translations are used whenever available. All other translations are my own. In all quotations, "ml/m^3" has been replaced by the synonymous designation "ppm."

2. On the degree of protection that the new value 0.1 mg/m^3 offers against cataracts, see the section on "Questionable Reporting."

3. For additional evidence, see in particular the section on "The Protection of Subpopulations."

4. In later years, irritation effects have sometimes been avoided for indirect reasons. In cases where (nongenotoxic) carcinogenicity is mediated by irritation, protection against irritation may yield protection against cancer. Hence, for vinyl acetate (1991), the commission said that the MAK value, being "oriented at the lowest irritation threshold for man," should protect against cancer as well. A similar statement was made about acetaldehyde (1986).

5. In German, *Leistungsfähigkeit* or *Arbeitsfähigkeit*.

6. Whereas so-called safety factors are adopted prior to decisions on individual substances, regulatory ratios are inferred *post factum*. When a decision has been based on a safety factor, the emerging regulatory ratio should be the inverse of the safety factor (e.g., if the safety factor is 100, then the regulatory ratio is 0.01). The quotient exposure limit/reference level was chosen for this purpose (rather than its inverse, reference level/exposure limit) partly to avoid confusions with safety (uncertainty) factors and partly to obtain a measure that is more intuitive when the exposure limit is higher than the reference level.

7. The commission referred to a WHO Expert Committee that recommended an acceptable daily intake (ADI) of 0.00003 mg amitrole per kilogram for humans. But "[f]or the workplace, however, other criteria and safety factors apply." The commission did not explain *why* safety factors should be three orders of magnitude smaller for occupational than for nonoccupational exposure. They did, however, refer to an article by Zielhuis and van der Kreek (1979). In arguing for small safety factors for occupational exposure, these authors emphasize that more health-protective practices are "not realistic for the present day society" (p. 200). Furthermore, since actual exposures to food additives are often considerably lower than the ADIs, the latter are "not always actually put to the test. However, such a systematic testing seems hardly possible to carry out in the general population, whereas occupational practice offers much better opportunities for putting to the test the acceptability of an extrapolation. Also for this reason, one may apply a smaller s[afety]. f[actor]. than in extrapolation to the general public" (p. 196). This appeal to techno-economic feasibility and, in particular, to the acceptability of using workers as guinea pigs clearly goes far beyond considerations of health.

8. The reduction in the MAK for ε-caprolactam mentioned above should perhaps be seen against the background that since 1972, the TLV had been 1 mg/m^3, only 1/25th of the previous German value.

9. For an alternative approach, see the section on "Statistical Evaluations" in Chapter 5.

10. On the significance of interspecies differences in respiration, see the section on "Animal Effect Levels."

CHAPTER 4. THE LOWEST VALUES

Most of this chapter is based on two published articles: "Swedish Occupational Exposure Limits—A Case Study in Administrative Risk Management," *Arbete Människa Miljö & Nordisk Ergonomi* (Luleå, Sweden) no 2, 1997, pp. 98–107 and "Critical Effects and Exposure Limits," *Risk Analysis* 17:227–236,

1997. (© Society for Risk Analysis). Thanks are due to the journals for allowing me to use this material.
 1. Geometric mean of all relevant ratios from the six lists covered by the period.
 2. The number of substances with an OEL rose from 75 in 1969 to 329 in 1994.
 3. References to the consensus reports are made by quoting the name of the substance and the year in which the report was adopted. The reports are all available in *Arbete och Hälsa* and can easily be located using the index published in that journal (Anon. 1994).
 4. It was not always clear how to categorize a given piece of information. An experimental result showing that a substance causes eye irritation in 1 out of 20 subjects at 7 ppm may be reported as a NEL (almost all subjects free from irritation effects at 7 ppm). Alternatively, it may be reported as an EL (one subject experienced eye irritation at 7 ppm). In cases like these, I have followed the NEL option if the committee's wording indicates that they see it that way; otherwise, the EL option is used.
 5. Some reports cover several related substances, and 14 substances have been the subject of more than one consensus report.
 6. From 1979 to 1984, 90 substances were reviewed, and to 39 of them (43%) a critical effect was assigned. From 1985 to 1989, 91 substances were reviewed and critical effects assigned to 80 (88%). From 1990 to the second half of 1994, 97 substances were reviewed and 56 (58%) were assigned a critical effect. A possible explanation of the declining frequency in later years is that, after having reported on most of the better-documented substances, the committee is now often dealing with substances for which very little toxicological information is available.
 7. On the reliability of this threshold, see the section on "The Quality of NEL_3."
 8. Morpholine, dust from polyvinyl chloride, nitromethane, acetonitrile, methyl formate, and wollastonite.
 9. These are ethyl benzene, ferric dimethyl dithiocarbamate, and 3-heptanone. For ethyl benzene, however, it was mentioned that 217 mg/m^3 caused behavioral disturbances in animals. The OEL is 200 mg/m^3.
 10. Ethylene glycol monopropyl ether, ethylene glycol monopropyl ether acetate, diethylene glycol, cathecol, hydroquinone, aniline, arsine, and nitrogen monoxide.
 11. 4,4'-Methylene dianiline, ethyl chloride, 1,2,3-trichlorobenzene, and 1,2,4-trichlorobenzene.
 12. *N,N*-Dimethylacetamide.
 13. The committee did not mention that in the same experiment 10 mg/m^3

caused "a slight but consistent increase" in the thickness of the cornea in two of four subjects (Ståhlbom et al. 1991). Concentrations below 10 mg/m³ were not tested. If this had been mentioned, an OEL/EL rate of 0.6 could have been calculated. As was pointed out to me by the committee's former chairman, Bo Holmberg, one of the experimenters was a member of the committee and probably contributed heavily to the decision on this substance.
14. Zinc dimethyl dithiocarbamate, propylene oxide, and chloroprene.
15. Disulfiram.
16. Thiram.
17. Chlorocresol.
18. Methyl mercaptan, dimethyl sulfide, and dimethyl disulfide.
19. For benzene, this was reported twice, in 1981 and 1988.

CHAPTER 5. SETTING BETTER STANDARDS

1. One reason this has not been much discussed may be that OELs have been incorrectly advertised as safe levels rather than as the outcome of compromises between health and economics.
2. Similar experiences have been reported from the Swedish OEL-setting process (Rudén 1997).
3. Muir (1988) reported that he had found it impossible to "trace the source and scientific basis" of the TLV for "nuisance dust." Its origins—but certainly no scientific basis—can be found in an article by Stokinger in which he recommended 5 mg/m³ since "it has been in satisfactory use for some years in controlling hematite dust and fume in at least one American plant" (Stokinger 1984 [1955] p. 76). In the same article, Stokinger said that it would be desirable to set a maximal limit of 1000 ppm for "most, although not all, of the gases and vapors that are apparently nontoxic or nonhazardous." This was the limit already set for "Freons and other apparently innocuous substances" (p. 74).
4. The lack of a general limit for volatiles, by analogy with the "nuisance value" of 5 mg/m³ for dusts, was pointed out by Gardner and Oldershaw (1990).
5. Body surface area is difficult to measure. It can, however, be estimated by the formula $a = k \times m^{2/3}$, where a denotes surface area and m body weight, and k is a constant. For doses to be approximately proportionate to body area it is sufficient that they are proportionate to body weight to the ⅔ power. Body weight to the ⅔ power is "an accepted surrogate for surface area" (Travis and White 1988, p. 120).
6. This is not the usual way of expressing the relationship. The conven-

tional method is to calculate the ratio of body weights and take its ⅔ power as a scaling factor without referring to the actual body surface areas.

7. Empirical studies indicate that metabolic rates increase with the ¾ power of body weight rather than with the ⅔ power. Therefore, some authors prefer the ¾ power of body weight as a scaling factor (Travis and White 1988, p. 14; Chappell 1989).

8. Even such an upper bound can, of course, only be inferred with reservations because of the possibility that the experiment was an improbable event.

9. The confidence level 0.95 in the definition of an OBEL has been chosen primarily because of the long-standing tradition in biostatistics to use this level for a wide variety of purposes. A case can be made for the use of higher confidence levels to minimize the risk of underestimating toxic effects. It may also be of interest to investigate, but more as a limiting case, a confidence level as low as 0.5. The definition of an OBEL can be modified to obtain variants such as $OBEL_{0.999}$ at the confidence level 0.999, $OBEL_{0.99}$ at the confidence level 0.99, and so on.

OBEL values are fairly insensitive to increased levels of confidence. (This can be seen from the shape of the relevant distributions, such as the normal distribution. Note, for instance, that $N_{0.999}/N_{0.95} \approx 1.9$.) As an example, suppose that an experiment shows no case of cancer in 150 animals exposed to 20 ppm of a substance. If the disease incidence at the experimental dose is p, then the probability of the obtained outcome is $(1 - p)^{150}$. This probability is 0.05 (i.e., the probability of a larger effect is 0.95) for the p such that $(1 - p)^{150} = 0.05$, i.e., for $p = 0.02$. Hence, 20 ppm is the OBEL(0.02) under the conditions of this experiment. With similar calculations we can show that 20 ppm = $OBEL_{0.999}(0.045)$ = $OBEL_{0.99}(0.03)$ = OBEL(0.02) = $OBEL_{0.5}(0.005)$.

Since the effect of raising the confidence level to values higher than 0.95 is small in relation to the wide variations in (the equally arbitrary) uncertainty factors, it does not seem reasonable, if one wishes to reduce risk taking, to focus on the former. The level 0.95 is defensible against this background.

10. Following the usual practice, the term *extrapolation* is used here for what is, strictly speaking, *inter*polation.

11. The OBEL is the solution of the equation $(1 - p)^{10} = 0.05$. Even if we choose the extremely liberal confidence limit 0.5, we obtain 10 ppm = $OBEL_{0.5}(0.07)$ and 1 ppm = $LEBEL_{0.5}(0.007)$.

APPENDIX: HOW TO COMPARE EXPOSURE LIMITS

1. This use of quotients relies in principle on a linear model of dose–response relationships. On the linearity assumption, see Chapter 5.

2. The number of substances on which the measures were based, i.e., the number of substances on the benchmark list with OELs on the respective lists, were as follows: Philippines 110, Turkey 111, United Kingdom 109, Australia 116, Germany 116, Japan 74, Finland 109, France 110, Denmark 117, Sweden 92, and Russia 96.

GLOSSARY

Adenocarcinoma carcinoma consisting of gland cells.

Aerosol suspension of small particles in the air.

Anemia shortage of red blood cells or of hemoglobin.

Angina pectoris pain in the breast caused by lack of oxygen in the heart muscle.

Antabuse effect a type of alcohol intolerance.

Argyria grayish discoloration of the skin due to silver.

Binocular affecting both eyes.

Bioactivation chemical transformation in the body that makes a substance more biologically active (more toxic).

Carboxyhemoglobin hemoglobin to which carbon monoxide has been bound, preventing it from carrying oxygen.

Carcinogenicity tendency to cause cancer.

Carcinoma malignant tumor that has grown out of epithelial cells (cells covering a surface).

Cataract clouding of the lens of the eye.

Cell culture growth of living cells outside of the body.

Chromosomes the parts of the cells that carry heredity and regulate cell division.

Chronaxy the time it takes for a nerve cell to react to an electrical stimulus.

Claudicatio intermittens pain in the legs provoked by walking and relieved by resting; generally caused by occlusive arterial disease.

Claudication lameness or limping.

CO-Hb proportion of the hemoglobin that has been transformed into carboxyhemoglobin.

Conjunctivitis inflammation of the conjunctiva (the thin mucous membrane that covers the inside of the eyelids and the front surface of the eyeball)

Creatinine a compound produced by the body and excreted in the urine. Its concentration in plasma is an indicator of the health status of the kidneys.

Cytogenetic pertaining to chromosomes and genes.

Cytolysis destruction and dissolution of cells.

Dermatitis inflammation of the skin.

Detoxification chemical transformation that makes a substance less toxic.

Diastolic blood pressure blood pressure during the phase in which the heart dilates, preparing for the next contraction.

DNA (deoxyribonucleic acid) the essential part of chromosomes.

Dose–effect relationship the relationship between the dose of a substance and its effects on exposed individual(s). It is defined for a substance.

Dose–response relationship the relationship between the dose of the substance and the frequency of the effect in a population. It is defined for a substance and an effect of that substance.

Edema   excessive fluid between the cells in a tissue.

Embryo   developing offspring at an early stage (in humans, up to 8 weeks).

Embryotoxic   toxic to the unborn child.

Endoplasmic reticulum   a fine microscopic system of folded membranes and interconnected small tubes in the cell.

Epithelioma   cancer that has grown out of epithelial cells (mainly skin and mucous membranes).

Epithelium   layer of cells that covers an internal or external surface of the body.

Erythrocyte   red blood cell.

Esthesioneuroepithelioma   cancer originating in the olfactory nerve.

Excretion   discharge from the body.

Fetus   developing offspring in the uterus (in humans, after 8 weeks; before that time it is called an *embryo*).

Fibrosis   abnormal formation of fibrous tissue.

f/ml   fibers per milliliter.

Free radical   a type of highly reactive molecule.

Gastritis   inflammation of the stomach.

Genotoxic   capable of damaging the DNA. Genotoxic substances may cause inheritable diseases.

Glucose tolerance   a measurement of the body's response to an oral dose of glucose. It is used in the diagnosis of diabetes.

Hemangioma   tumor consisting of blood vessels.

Hemoglobin   the oxygen-carrying molecule in red blood cells.

Hemolytic   causing hemoglobin to be released from the red blood cells into the plasma.

Hepatic   pertaining to the liver.

Hepatocellular   pertaining to liver cells.

Histopathology   the microscopic study of diseased tissues.

Hyperplasia   abnormal growth of normal cells.

Hypertension   excessively high blood pressure.

Hypotension   excessively low blood pressure.

LC50 (LC_{50})   median lethal concentration, the concentration that kills half of the animals under experimental conditions.

Leukemia   malignant growth of white blood cells (leukocytes) and their precursors in the blood and in the spleen, lymphatic glands, and bone marrow.

Leukocytosis   excessive number of leukocytes (white blood cells).

LOAEL   (lowest observed adverse effect level) lowest dose or exposure level at which an adverse effect has been observed.

Lymphoid   pertaining to lymph or lymphatic tissue.

Malignancy   the quality of being malignant; malignant tumor (cancer).

Mammary   pertaining to the (female) breast.

Metabolism   the sum of chemical processes that maintain a living organism. The metabolism of a foreign substance in the body is the pattern of chemical transformations to which it is subject.

Metabolite   substance produced by the body's own chemical reactions.

Methemoglobin   a dysfunctional form of hemoglobin that is incapable of transporting oxygen.

Micronucleus   a type of dense, round structure that is found in most cells.

ml/m^3   milliliters per cubic meter (the same as ppm).

mppcf   million particles per cubic foot.

Narcotic   producing sleep or drowsiness.

Neoplasia   abnormal growth, tumor.

Neurasthenia   abnormal fatigability and lack of mental energy.

Neurotoxic   toxic to the nervous system.

Nictitating membrane a folded mucous membrane that can be drawn over the eye, functioning as a third eyelid. It is present in reptiles, birds, and some mammals.

Organogenesis formation of organs.

Palpitation fast or irregular heartbeats.

Paralysis loss of feeling, of the ability to move, or both.

Parenchymatous pertaining to the parenchyma, the characteristic functional tissue of an organ.

Parkinson's disease a neurological disease characterized by muscular rigidity and tremor of the hands.

Pathogenic producing disease.

Peribronchitis inflammation of the tissues surrounding the bronchi.

Pharmacokinetics the study of the absorption, tissue distribution, metabolism, and excretion of drugs.

Plasma the fluid part of the blood (except for the blood cells).

Pneumonia inflammation of the lungs.

Polyneuritis inflammation of many nerves.

Polyneuropathy disease that affects many nerves.

ppb parts per billion.

ppm parts per million.

Prenatal before birth.

Proliferation growth through multiplication of cells.

Pulmonary pertaining to the lung.

Punctate resembling points.

Renal pertaining to the kidneys.

Reticulocytosis excessive number of reticulocytes (immature red blood cells).

Rhinitis inflammation of the membranes of the nose.

Scaling factor a factor used to translate a toxic dose between species with different body sizes.

Sedative   calming or putting to sleep.

Sputum   matter originating in the lung, from which it has been transported to the mouth.

Squamous cell carcinoma   a type of cancer that can be found in several different organs. The most common type of lung cancer is a squamous cell carcinoma.

Subacute   between chronic and acute but closer to the latter.

Subchronic   between chronic and acute but closer to the former.

Subnarcotic   weakly narcotic.

Systemic   affecting the body as a whole.

Systolic blood pressure   blood pressure during the phase in which the heart contracts and forces blood into the arteries.

Teratogenic   causing physical defects in the unborn child.

Testis   (plural: *testes*) testicle.

Thrombocytopenia   shortage of blood platelets.

Tissue culture   growth of a tissue outside of the body.

Trace quantity   very small quantity.

Tubular   pertaining to tubules (e.g., the tubules of the kidney, from which the urine flows via the ureter into the bladder).

Vegetative nervous system   (autonomic nervous system) the part of the nervous system that regulates blood vessels, secretory glands, and internal organs.

Vestibule   cavity. The vestibule of the ear is a cavity in the middle of the bony labyrinth.

Vitiligo   white patches on the skin (without melanin pigment).

Volatile   liquid with a strong tendency to evaporate.

REFERENCES

ACGIH (1996). *1996 TLVs and BEIs*. Cincinnati, American Conference of Governmental Industrial Hygienists.
ACGIH, Board of Directors (1990). "Threshold Limit Values: A More Balanced Appraisal." *Appl Occup Environ Hyg* 5: 340–344.
Adkins, C. F., et al (1990). "To the Editor." *Appl Occup Environ Hyg* 5: 748–750.
Ahlborg, U. G., H. Håkanson, F. Wærn, and A. Hanberg (1988). *Nordisk dioxinriskbedömning. Rapport från en nordisk expertgrupp, NORD 1988:49*. Copenhagen, Nordisk Ministerråd.
Ambrose, A. M. (1950). "Toxicological Studies of Compounds Investigated for Use as Inhibitors of Biological Processes II. Toxicity of Ethylene Chlorohydrin." *Arch Industr Hyg Occup Med* 2: 591–597.
Andersson, A. (1957). *Gesundheitliche Gefahren in der Industrie bei Exposition für Trichloräthylen. Acta Med Scand Suppl 323*.
Anon. (1994). "Consensus Reports in Previous Volumes." *Arbete och hälsa* 1994 (30): 68–72.
ASS (1993). "Hygieniska gränsvärden" ["Occupational Exposure Limits"].

Arbetarskyddsstyrelsens författningssamling, AFS, 1993:9. Stockholm, Arbetarskyddsstyrelsen.
Bailar, J. C., E.A.C. Crouch, R. Shaikh, and D. Spiegelman (1988). "One-Hit Models of Carcinogenesis: Conservative or Not?" *Risk Analysis* 8: 485–497.
Bailar, J. C., E. A. C. Crouch, D. Spiegelman, and R. Shaikh (1990). "Response to Park." *Risk Analysis* 10: 211–212.
Booth, C. C. (1993). "Clinical Research." Pp. 205–229 in W. F. Bynum and R. Porter (eds.), *Companion Encyclopedia of the History of Medicine*. London, Routledge.
Breysse, P. (1991). "ACGIH TLVs: A Critical Analysis of the Documentation." *Am J Industr Med* 20: 423–428.
Brieger, H., and W. A. Hodes (1951). "Toxic Effects of Exposure to Vapors of Aliphatic Amines." *AMA Arch Industr Hyg Occup Med* 3: 287–291.
Brown, K. G., and L. S. Erdreich (1989). "Statistical Uncertainty in the No-Observed-Adverse-Effect Level." *Fundamental Appl Toxicol* 13: 235–244.
Carter, V. L. (1985). "Modus Operandi of Committee on Threshold Limit Values for Chemical Substances." *Ann Am Conf Govern Industr Hygienists* 12: 11–13.
Castleman, B. I., and G. E. Ziem (1988). "Corporate Influence on Threshold Limit Values." *Am J Industr Med* 13: 531–559.
Catalano, P. J., and L. M. Ryan (1994). "Statistical Issues in Developmental Toxicology." Pp. 123–136 in C. M. Smith, D. C. Christiani, and K. T. Kelsey (eds.), *Chemical Risk Assessment and Occupational Health*. London, Auburn House.
Chappell, W. R. (1989). "Interspecific Scaling of Toxicity Data: A Question of Interpretation." *Risk Analysis* 9: 13–14.
Cook, W. A. (1985). "History of ACGIH TLVs." *Ann Am Conf Govern Industr Hygienists* 12: 3–9.
Cook, W. A. (1987). *Occupational Exposure Limits—Worldwide*. Akron, OH, American Industrial Hygiene Association.
Cox, G. V. (1991). "Comments on 'Implications of OSHA's Reliance on TLVs in Developing the Air Contaminants Standard'." *Am J Industr Med* 20: 823–824.
Crawford, M., and R. Wilson (1996) "Low-Dose Linearity: The Rule or the Exception." *Hum Ecol Risk Assess* 2: 305–330.
Crump, K. S. (1984). "A New Method for Determining Allowable Daily Intakes." *Fundamental Appl Toxicol* 4: 854–871.
Cullen, M. R. (1991). "Implications for the Use of TLVs to Clinical Occupational Medicine Practice." *Am J Industr Med* 19: 679–680.

De Renzo, D. J. (1986). *Solvents Safety Handbook.* Park Ridge, NJ, Noyes Data Corporation.

DFG (1991–1994). *Occupational Toxicants. Critical Data Evaluation for MAK Values and Classification of Carcinogens, Parts 1–6.* Weinheim, Deutsche Forschungsgemeinschaft.

Dietl, J. (1849). *Der Aderlass in der Lungenentzündung.* Vienna, Kaulfuss Witwe, Prandel & Comp.

Djuric, D. (1988). "Comments on the Article by Castleman and Ziem." *Am J Industr Med* 13: 613–614.

Dror, K. (1988). "TLVs—A Personal Opinion." *Am J Industr Med* 13: 617–618.

Ebner, H., M. Helletzgruber, R. Höfer, H. Kolbe, M. Weissel, and N. Winker (1979). "Vitiligo Durch *p*-tert. Butylphenol." *Dermatosen Beruf Umwelt* 27: 99–104.

Egilman, D. S. (1992). "Public Health and Epistemology." *Am J Industr Med* 22: 457–459.

Feiner, B., W. J. Burke, and J. Baliff (1946). "An Industrial Hygiene Survey of an Onion Dehydrating Plant." *J Industr Hyg Toxicol* 28: 278–279.

Finkel, A. M. (1994). "The Case for 'Plausible Conservatism' in Choosing and Altering Defaults." Pp. 601–627 in National Research Council, *Science and Judgment in Risk Assessment.* Washington DC, National Academy Press.

Freiman, J. A., T. C. Chalmers, H. Smith, and R. R. Kuebler (1978). "The Importance of Beta, the Type II Error and Sampe Size in the Design and Interpretation of the Randomized Control Trial." *N Engl J Med* 299: 690–694.

Gardner, R. J., and P. J. Oldershaw (1990). "Development of Pragmatic Exposure-Control Concentrations Based on Packaging Regulation Risk Phrases." *Ann Occup Hyg* 35: 51–59.

Gillette, J. R., and R. W. Estabrook (1987). "Evaluation of Xenobiotic Metabolism." Pp. 357–374 in R. G. Tardiff and J. V. Rodricks (eds.), *Toxic Substances and Human Risk.* New York, Plenum Press.

Golz, H. H., B. D. Culver, H. L. Hardy, L. H. Miller, R. L. Raleigh, G. Roush, and T. W. Tusing (1966). "Report of an Investigation of Threshold Limit Values and Their Usage." *J Occup Med* 8: 280–283.

Grandjean, E., R. Münchinger, V. Turrian, P. A. Haas, H. K. Knoepfel, and H. Rosenmund (1955). "Investigations into the Effects of Exposure to Trichloroethylene in Mechanical Engineering." *Br J Industr Med* 12: 131–142.

Hagmar, L., T. Bellander, B. Bergöö, and B. G. Simonsson (1982). "Piperazine-Induced Occupational Asthma." *J Occup Med* 24: 193–197.

Hansson, S. O. (1982). *Acceptabel risk? Om gränsvärden i arbetsmiljön [Acceptable Risk? On Exposure Limits in the Working Environment]*. Stockholm, Tiden.

Hansson, S. O. (1989). "Dimensions of Risk." *Risk Analysis* 9: 107–112.

Hansson, S. O. (1993a). "Entscheidungsfindung bei Uneinigkeit der Experten." Pp. 87–96 in H. Zilleβen, P. C. Dienel, and W. Strubelt (eds.), *Die Modernisierung der Demokratie, Internationale Ansätze*. Opladen, Westdeutscher Verlag.

Hansson, S. O. (1993b). "The False Promises of Risk Analysis." *Ratio* 6: 16–26.

Hansson, S. O. (1995). "The Detection Level." *Regul Toxicol Pharmacol* 22: 103–109.

Hansson, S. O. (1996). "Decision-Making Under Great Uncertainty." *Philos Soc Sci* 26: 369–386.

Hansson, S. O. (1997a). "Can We Reverse the Burden of Proof?" *Toxicol Lett* 90: 223–228.

Hansson, S. O. (1997b). "Critical Effects and Exposure Limits." *Risk Analysis* 17:227–236.

Hansson, S. O. (1997c). "What Is Philosophy of Risk?" *Theoria*, in press.

Hansson, S. O., and M. Johannesson (1997). "Decision-Theoretic Approaches to Global Climate Change." Pp. 153–178 in G. Fermann (ed.), *The Politics of Climate Change*. Oslo, Scandinavian University Press.

Henschler, D. (1984). "Exposure Limits: History, Philosophy, Future Developments." *Ann Occup Hyg* 28: 79–92.

Henschler, D. (1991). "The Concept of Occupational Exposure Limits." *Sci Total Environ* 101: 9–16.

Jellinek, S. D. (1981). "On the Inevitability of Being Wrong." *Annals NY Acad Sci* 363: 43–47.

Keplinger, M. L., J. W. Goode, D. E. Gordon, and J. C. Calandra (1975). "Interim Results of Exposure of Rats, Hamsters, and Mice to Vinyl Chloride." *Ann NY Acad Sci* 246: 219–220.

Kramer, C. G., and J. E. Mutchler (1972). "The Correlation of Clinical and Environmental Measurements for Workers Exposed to Vinyl Chloride." *Am Industr Hyg Assoc J* 33: 19–30.

Krewski, D., M. J. Goddard, and D. Murdoch (1989). "Statistical Considerations in the Interpretation of Negative Carcinogenicity Data." *Regul Toxicol Pharmacol* 9: 5–22.

LaNier, M. E. (1984). *Threshold Limit Values—Discussion and Thirty-five Year Index with Recommendations. Annals of the American Conference of Governmental Industrial Hygienists*, vol. 9. Cincinnati, ACGIH.

Lauwerys, R. R. (1991). "Re: 'OSHA's Reliance on TLVs'." *Am J Industr Med* 19: 827.

Lauwerys, R. R., A. Kivits, M. Lhoir, P. Rigolet, D. Houbeau, J. P. Buchet, and H. A. Roels (1980). "Biological Surveillance of Workers Exposed to Dimethylformamide and the Influence of Skin Protection on Its Percutaneous Absorption." *Int Arch Occup Environ Health* 44: 189–203.

Lee, J. S. (1987). "A Message from the Chair of ACGIH." *Appl Industr Hyg* 2: F6–F7.

Leisenring, W., and L. Ryan (1992). "Statistical Properties of the NOAEL." *Regul Toxicol Pharmacol* 15: 161–171.

Leung, H. W., and D. Paustenbach (1988). "Setting Occupational Exposure Limits for Irritant Organic Acids and Bases Based on Their Equilibrium Dissociation Constants." *Appl Industr Hyg* 3: 115–118.

Levi, I. (1962). "On the Seriousness of Mistakes." *Philos Sci* 29: 47–65.

Lichtenstein, M. E., F. Bartl, and R. T. Pierce (1975). "Control of Cobalt Exposures during Wet Process Tungsten Carbide Grinding." *Am Industr Hyg Assoc J* 36: 879–885.

Lundberg, P., and B. Holmberg (1985). "Occupational Standard Setting in Sweden—Procedure and Criteria." *Ann Am Conf Govern Industr Hyg* 12: 249–252.

Lundberg, P., A. Löf, G. Johanson, A. Wennberg, J. Högberg, and B. Holmberg (1991). "New Swedish Occupational Standards for Some Organic Solvents." *Am J Industr Med* 19: 559–567.

Magnuson, H. (1965). "Soviet and American Standards for Industrial Health." *Arch Environ Health* 10: 542–545.

Maltoni, C., and G. Lefemine (1975). "Carcinogenicity Bioassays of Vinyl Chloride: Current Results." *Ann NY Acad Sci* 246: 195–218.

Maltoni, C., G. Lefemine, A. Ciliberti, G. Cotti, and D. Carretti (1981). "Carcinogenicity Bioassays of Vinyl Chloride Monomer: A Model of Risk Assessment on an Experimental Basis." *Environ Health Perspect* 41: 3–29.

Maltoni, C., G. Lefemine, G. Cotti, P. Chieco, and V. Patella (1985). *Experimental Research on Vinylidene Chloride Carcinogenesis*. C. Maltoni and M. A. Mehlman (eds.), *Archives of Research on Industrial Carcinogenesis*, vol. III. Princeton, NJ, Princeton Scientific Publishers.

Marshall, E. (1983). "Federal Court Finds IBT Officials Guilty of Fraud." *Science* 222: 488.

Mastromatteo, E. (1981). "On the Concept of Threshold." *Am Industr Hyg Assoc J* 42: 763–770.

Miller, R. W. (1978). "The Discovery of Human Teratogens, Carcinogens and Mutagens." Pp. 101–126 in A. Hollaender and F. J. DeSerres (eds.),

Chemical Mutagens—Priorities and Mechanisms for Their Detection, vol. 5. New York, Plenum Press.

Morgan, R. W. (1992). "Attitudes About Asbestos and Lung Cancer." *Am J Industr Med* 22: 437–441.

Morton, W. E. (1988). "The Nature and Significance of the Corporate Influence on Threshold Limit Values." *Am J Industr Med* 14: 721–723.

Muir, D.C.F. (1988). "TLVs—What Now?" *Am J Industr Med* 13: 605–606.

Myers, J. E. (1991). "Re: Implications of OSHA's Reliance on TLVs in Developing the Air Contaminants Standard." *Am J Industr Med* 19: 832–834.

National Research Council (NRC) (1994). *Science and Judgment in Risk Assessment*. Washington, DC, National Academy Press.

Nicholson, W. J. (1981). "Criteria Document for Swedish Occupational Standards: Asbestos and Inorganic Fibers." *Arbete och hälsa* 1981: 17.

Nordberg, G. F., H. Frostling, P. Lundberg, and P. Westerholm (1988). "Swedish Occupational Exposure Limits: Developments in Scientific Evaluation and Documentation." *Am J Industr Med* 14: 217–221.

Park, C. N. (1990). " 'Underestimation' of Linear Models." *Risk Analysis* 10: 209–210.

Paull, J. M. (1984). "The Origin and Basis of Threshold Limit Values." *Am J Industr Med* 5: 227–238.

Paustenbach, D. J. (1997). "OSHA's Program for Updating the Permissible Exposure Limits (PELs): Can Risk Assessment Help 'Move the Ball Forward'?" *Risk Perspect* (Harvard Center for Risk Analysis) 5(1): 1–6.

Paxman, D. G. and J. C. Robinson (1990). "Regulation of Occupational Carcinogens under OSHA's Air Contaminants Standard." *Regul Toxicol Pharmacol* 12: 296–308.

Peters, P.W.J., and J. M. Garbis-Berkvens (1996). "General Reproductive Toxicology." Pp. 929–946 in R. J. Niesink, J. de Vries, and M. A. Hollinger (eds.), *Toxicology. Principles and Applications*. Boca Raton, FL, CRC Press.

Pfeiffer, K. P., and T. Kenner (1986). "The Risk Concept in Medicine." *Theor Med* 7: 259–268.

Pinkel, D. (1958). "The Use of Body Surface Area as a Criterion of Drug Dosage in Cancer Chemotherapy." *Cancer Res* 18: 853–856.

Pohl, H. R., and H. G. Abadin (1995). "Utilizing Uncertainty Factors in Minimal Risk Levels Derivation." *Regul Toxicol Pharmacol* 22: 180–188.

Rappaport, S. M. (1993). "Threshold Limit Values, Permissible Exposure Limits, and Feasibility: The Basis for Exposure Limits in the United States." *Am J Industr Med* 23: 683–694.

Richter, E. D. (1988). "On 'Corporate Influence on Threshold Limit Values' by Castleman and Ziem." *Am J Industr Med* 14: 365–368.

Roach, S. A., and S. M. Rappaport (1990). "But They Are Not Thresholds: A Critical Analysis of the Documentation of Threshold Limit Values." *Am J Industr Med* 17: 727–753.

Robinson, J. C., and D. G. Paxman (1992). "The Role of Threshold Limit Values in U.S. Air Pollution Policy." *Am J Industr Med* 21: 383–396.

Robinson, J. C., D. G. Paxman, and S. M. Rappaport (1991). "Implications of OSHA's Reliance on TLVs in Developing the Air Contaminants Standard." *Am J Industr Med* 19: 3–13.

Rudén, C. (1997) *Hur sätts svenska gränsvärden?* [*How Are Swedish Exposure Limits Decided*?], mimeographed. Uppsala, Uppsala University, Department of Philosophy.

Rudner, R. (1953). "The Scientist Qua Scientist Makes Value Judgments." *Philos Sci* 20: 1–6.

Ruth, J. H. (1986). "Odor Thresholds and Irritation Levels of Several Chemical Substances: A Review." *Am Industr Hyg Assoc J* 47: A142–A151.

Salter, L. (1988). *Mandated Science: Science and Scientists in the Making of Standards*. Dordrecht, Kluwer Academic Publishers.

Savolainen, H., R. Tenhunen, and H. Härkönen (1985). "Reticulocyte Haem Synthesis in Occupational Exposure to Trinitrotoluene." *Br J Industr Med* 42: 354–355.

Savolainen, K., V. Riihimäki, A. M. Seppäläinen, and M. Linnoila (1980). "Effects of Short-Term *m*-Xylene Exposure and Physical Exercise on the Central Nervous System." *Int Arch Occup Environ Health* 45: 105–121.

Schultz, W. B. (1988). "Why the FDA's De Minimis Interpretation of the Delaney Clause Is a Violation of Law." *J Am College Toxicol* 7: 521–527.

Senatskommission zur Prüfung gesundheitsschädlicher Arbeitsstoffe (1995). *Gesundheitsschädliche Arbeitsstoffe: Toxikologisch-arbeitsmedizinische Begründungen von MAK-Werten (Maximale Arbeitsplatzkonzentrationen)*, 1.–21. Lieferung. Weinheim, Deutsche Forschungsgemeinschaft.

Senatskommission zur Prüfung gesundheitsschädlicher Arbeitsstoffe (1996a). *List of MAK and BAT Values 1996*. Weinheim, Deutsche Forschungsgemeinschaft.

Senatskommission zur Prüfung gesundheitsschädlicher Arbeitsstoffe (1996b). *MAK- und BAT-Werte-Liste 1996*. Weinheim, Deutsche Forschungsgemeinschaft.

Sentes, R. (1989). "Occupational Exposure Standards in Canada: From ACGIH to?" *Am J Industr Med* 16: 719–722.

Sentes, R. (1992). "OSHA and Standard-Setting." *Am J Industr Health* 21: 759–764.
Sielken, R. L. (1990). "Driving Cancer Dose–Response Modeling with Data, Not Assumptions." *Risk Analysis* 10: 207–208.
Ståhlbom, B., T. Lundh, I. Florén, and B. Åkesson (1991). "Visual Disturbances in Man as a Result of Experimental and Occupational Exposure to Dimethylethylamine." *Br J Industr Med* 48: 26–29.
Stokinger, H. E. (1963). "International Threshold Limit Values—1963." *Am Industr Hyg Assoc J* 24: 469–474.
Stokinger, H. E. (1969). "Current Problems of Setting Occupational Exposure Standards." *Arch Environ Health* 19: 277–281.
Stokinger, H. E. (1984). "The Case for Carcinogen TLVs Continues Strong." *Ann Am Conf Govern Industr Hygienists* 9: 257–264.
Stokinger, H. E. (1984 [1955]). "Standards for Safeguarding the Health of the Industrial Worker." *Ann Am Conf Govern Industr Hygienists* 9: 73–82.
Stokinger, H. E. (1984 [1956]). "Prepared Discussion." *Ann Am Conf Govern Industr Hygienists* 9: 88–91.
Stokinger, H. E. (1984 [1981]). "Threshold Limit Values." *Ann Am Conf Govern Industr Hygienists* 9: 275–281.
Stokinger, H. E. (1987). "Nonstatistical vs. Illusory Statistical Approaches to the Estimation of Risk from Environmental Chemicals." *Dangerous Properties Industr Materials Rep* 7: 2–8.
Stokinger, H. E. (1988). "Threshold Limit Values: Any Alternative?" *Am J Industr Med* 14: 231–232.
Takamatsu, M. (1962). "Health Hazards in Workers Exposed to Trichloroethylene Vapor II." *Kumamoto Med J* 15: 43–54.
Travis, C. C., and R. K. White (1988). "Interspecific Scaling of Toxicity Data." *Risk Analysis* 8: 119–125.
Treon, J. F., W. E. Crutchfield, and K. V. Kitzmiller (1943). "The Physiological Response of Animals to Cyclohexane, Methylcyclohexane, and Certain Derivatives of These Compounds. II Inhalation." *J Industr Hyg Toxicol* 25: 323–347.
Tsuchiya, K. (1988). "Significance and Use of Threshold Limit Values with Reference to 'Corporate Influence on Threshold Limit Values' by Castleman and Ziem." *Am J Industr Med* 14: 215–216.
Vainio, H., and L. Tomatis (1985). "Exposure to Carcinogens: Scientific and Regulatory Aspects." *Ann Am Conf Govern Industr Hygienists* 12: 135–143.
Vladeck, D. C., and S. M. Wolfe (1991). "The Politics of OSHA's Standard-Setting." *Am J Industr Med* 19: 801–804.
Watanabe, P. G., R. E. Hefner, and P. J. Gehring (1976). "Vinyl Chloride–

Induced Depression of Hepatic Non-protein Sulfhydryl Content and Effects on Bromosulphalein (BSP) Clearance in Rats.'' *Toxicology* 6: 1–8.

Webster, I. (1989). ''Re: Corporate Influence on the Threshold Limit Values.'' *Am J Industr Med* 15: 121.

Wedeen, R. P. (1991). ''TLVs and the Contribution of Science to Policy.'' *Am J Industr Med* 19: 684–685.

Weeks, J. L., B. S. Levy, and G. R. Wagner (1991). *Preventing Occupational Disease and Injury*. Washington, DC, American Public Health Association.

Weinberg, A. M. (1972). ''Science and Trans-Science.'' *Minerva* 10: 209–222.

Wilkinson, L. (1993). ''Epidemiology.'' Pp. 1262–1282 in W. Bynum and R. Porter (eds.), *Companion Encyclopaedia of the History of Medicine*, vol. 2. London, Routledge.

Woitowitz, H. J. (1988). ''Maximum Concentrations at the Workplace in the Federal Republic of Germany.'' *Am J Industr Med* 14: 223–229.

Zeiger, E. (1987). ''Carcinogenicity of Mutagens: Predictive Capability of the Salmonella Mutagenesis Assay for Rodent Carcinogenicity.'' *Cancer Res* 47: 1287–1296.

Zenz, C., and B. A. Berg (1967). ''Human Responses to Controlled Vanadium Pentoxide Exposure.'' *Arch Environ Health* 14: 709–712.

Zielhuis, R. L., and F. W. van der Kreek (1979). ''The Use of a Safety Factor in Setting Health Based Permissible Levels for Occupational Exposure.'' *Int Arch Occup Environ Health* 42: 191–201.

Zielhuis, R. L., and A.A.E. Wibowo (1989). ''Standard Setting in Occupational Health: 'Philosophical' Issues.'' *Am J Industr Med* 16: 569–598.

Zielhuis, R. L., and A.A.E. Wibowo (1991). ''Alternative Sources of TLVs.'' *Am J Industr Med* 19: 830–831.

Ziem, G. E., and B. I. Castleman (1989). ''Threshold Limit Values: Historical Perspectives and Current Practice.'' *J Occup Med* 31: 910–918.

INDEX

Acceptable daily intake, 85, 136n. 7
Acetaldehyde, 40, 86, 128, 135n. 4
Acetic acid, 86–88, 128
Acetone, 40, 84, 128
Acetonitrile, 137n. 8
Acetylene dichloride, 129
ACGIH, 13, 17–34. *See also* TLVs
Acrolein, 128
Acrylonitrile, 128
ADI, 85, 136n. 7
Adjacent-list method, 124
Affirming the consequent, 30
Agent Orange, 58
Aggregation level, 106–9
Air pollution standards, 20
Allowable daily intake, 85, 136n. 7
Allyl alcohol, 86
Allyl chloride, 93
Allyl propyl disulfide, 40
Aluminum, 89
American Conference of Governmental Industrial Hygienists, 13, 17–34. *See also* TLVs
American Standards Association, 18
Amitrole, 50–52
Ammonia, 86, 128
Amyl acetate, 86, 126, 128
Angina pectoris, 44
Angiosarcoma, 32
Aniline, 128, 137n. 10
Animal experiments, 4–7, 11–12
Antimony trihydride, 131
Argentina, 19
Argyria, 95
Aristotle, 30

Arithmetic mean, 123
Arsenic, 97
Arsenic hydride, 128
Arsine, 128, 137n. 10
ASA, 18
Asbestos, 4, 22, 96–97
Asthma, 88–89
Asymmetry, epistemic, 11–12
Atrazine, 54, 58
Attapulgite, 91
Australia, 13–14, 19, 140n. 2
Austria, 19
Average, 123
  time-weighted, 126–27
Azinphos-methyl, 54, 57

Bacteria, 6
Barium peroxide, 128
Base-year method, 124
BAT, 35, 46
Belgium, 19
Benchmark list, 124–31
Benzene, 24–25, 96, 98, 107, 128, 138n. 19
Benzoquinone, 66–67
Beryllium, 28
Bioactivation, 4, 6
Biological monitoring, 35
Birth defects, 46, 94. *See also* embryotoxic effects and genotoxicity
Bis(2-chloroethyl)ether, 129
BL quotient, 127
Blood, 82, 93
Bloodletting, 2
Body surface area, 112, 138–39
Body weight, 112
Bounded effect levels, 114–17
Brazil, 19
Britain, 13–14, 19, 140n. 2

Bromine, 128
Bromomethane, 130
Burden of proof, 8–12, 111
Butadiene, 128
Butanol, 86, 128
Butanone, 130
Butoxydiglycol, 53–55
Butoxyethanol, 59, 128
Butyl acetate, 86, 128
Butyl acrylate, 64–65
Butyl alcohol, 86, 128
Butyl cellosolve, 128
Butylphenol, 50–51

Cadmium, 25, 93–94, 128
Canada, 19
Cancer, 9, 11, 32, 36, 76–78, 96–98
Caprolactam, 50–53, 84, 136n. 8
Carbon dioxide, 128
Carbon disulfide, 29, 41, 128
Carbon monoxide, 44, 128
Carbon tetrachloride, 128
Carcinogens, 9, 11, 32, 36, 76–78, 96–98
Carney, Thomas, 9
Carter, Vernon, 25
Case reports, 3
Castleman, Barry, 24, 26
Cathecol, 137n. 10
Ceiling values, 18, 86, 126–27
Cell cultures, 6
Cellosolve, 128
Cellosolve acetate, 128
Central nervous system, 6, 82, 91–93
Chemicals level, 106
Chile, 19
Chlorine, 60–61, 128

Chloroacetic acid methyl ester, 54, 57, 68, 116
Chloro-bensylidene malonitrile, 86
Chlorobenzene, 130
Chlorobutadiene, 128
Chlorocresol, 138n. 17
Chloroethanol, 129
Chloroform, 61–62, 128
Chloromethane, 54, 56
Chloro nitropropane, 128
Chloroprene, 54–55, 128, 138n. 14
Chromates, 28, 126
Chromic acid, 126, 128
Chromium, 97–98
Chronaxy, 30
Clinical tests, 2–3
Coal dust, 90
Cobalt, 89, 99, 101
Combination effects, 22
Compensation claims, 20
Compromise, economical, 15, 23, 35–37, 42–43, 46, 76, 103–10, 119–20, 136n. 7
Confidence level, 139n. 9
Consensus, 121–22
Consensus reports, 76, 78–80, 82, 121
Consequent, affirming, 30
Conservativity, interpretative, 110–13
Corneal edema, 94
Corporate information, 27–29, 76
Cost effectiveness, 107
Costs, 15, 23, 35–37, 42–43, 46, 76, 103–10, 119–20, 136n. 7
Cotton dust, 90
Criteria group, 76, 78–82, 121
Critical effect, 47, 81–82, 96, 137n. 6
Critical level, 96

Cyclohexane, 49–50, 68, 128
Cyclohexanol, 128
Cyclohexanone, 86, 128
Cyclohexene, 128

2,4-D, 54, 58
Default values, 108
Denmark, 13–14, 19, 140n. 2
DES (diethylstilbestrol), 9
Detection level, 113–14
Detoxification, 4
Diacetone alcohol, 86
Dichlorobenzene, 60–61, 128
Dichlorodifluoromethane, 128
Dichloroethane, 129
Dichloroethylene, 129
Dichloroethyl ether, 129
Dichlorofluoromethane, 129
Dichloromethane, 129
Dichloromonofluoromethane, 129
Dichloronitroethane, 128
Dichlorotetrafluoroethane, 126, 128
Dicyclopentadiene, 86
Diethylamine, 61–62
Diethylene glycol, 59, 137n. 10
Diethylene glycol dimethyl ether, 54, 57
Diethyl ether, 129
Diethylstilbestrol, 9
Dietl, Joseph, 2
Diisocyanates, 29, 88, 90
Diisopropyl ether, 130
Dimethylacetamide, 137n. 12
Dimethylamine, 61, 63, 65
Dimethylaniline, 126, 129
Dimethyl disulfide, 138n. 18
Dimethyl ether, 54–55
Dimethylethylamine, 94
Dimethylformamide, 46, 50–52, 99–101

Dimethyl sulfate, 129
Dimethyl sulfide, 138n. 18
Dinitrotoluene, 94, 126, 129
Dioxane, 86, 126, 129
Dipropylene glycol monomethyl ether, 85, 100–101
Discomfort. *See* irritation effects
Disulfiram, 138n. 15
DNA, 7
Documentation of OELs, 14–15, 18, 24, 27, 35, 76, 81, 102, 110
Dow Chemical Company, 31–32
Drugs, 109

Economical feasibility, 15, 23, 35–37, 42–43, 46, 76, 103–10, 119–20, 136n. 7
EL, 82
Embryotoxicity, 45–47, 94–95. *See also* Genotoxicity
Environmental Protection Agency (EPA), 111
EPA, 111
Epidemiology, 3–4, 7, 12–13, 29
Epistemic asymmetry, 11–12
Erionite, 96
Errors (types I and II), 7–11, 113
Ethanol, 86, 129
Ether, ethyl, 86–87, 129
Ethoxyethanol, 128
Ethoxyethyl acetate, 128
Ethyl acetate, 86, 129
Ethyl acrylate, 59, 65
Ethyl alcohol, 86, 129
Ethylamine, 61, 63
Ethyl benzene, 61–62, 129, 137n. 9
Ethyl bromide, 129
Ethyl chloride, 129, 137n. 11
Ethylene chlorohydrine, 71, 129

Ethylene dichloride, 129
Ethylene glycol, 86
Ethylene glycol dinitrate, 43
Ethylene glycol monomethyl ether, 130
Ethylene glycol monomethyl ether acetate, 130
Ethylene glycol monopropyl ether, 137n. 10
Ethylene glycol monopropyl ether acetate, 137n. 10
Ethylene oxide, 97, 129
Ethyl ether, 86–87, 129
Ethyl formate, 129
Ethyl glycol, 94–95
Ethylidene chloride, 129
Ethylidene dichloride, 129
Ethyl silicate, 129
Exception values, 108–9
Experiments, 3
  on animals, 4–7, 11–12
  on humans, 3, 22
Experts, 120–22
Exposure chambers, 22
Exposure limits. *See* OELs
Extrapolation, 6, 110, 139n. 10
  linear, 115–17
Eye, 94

Fairhall, L.T., 28
False negative, 7
False positive, 7
Falsificationism, 12
Female workers, 45–47
Fenthion, 54, 57
Ferric dimethyl dithiocarbamate, 137n. 9
Fetotoxicity, 45–47, 94–95. *See also* Genotoxicity
Filing procedures, 27

Finland, 13–14, 140n. 2
Fluorides, 30, 126, 129
Food additives, 109
Formaldehyde, 86, 129
France, 13–14, 140n. 2
Free radicals, 32
Freon, 53, 60, 94, 128–30, 138n. 3
Furfural, 86
Furfuryl alcohol, 54–56

Gender, 45–47
Genetic variability, 5
Genotoxicity, 36, 95
 tests, 6–7
Geometric mean, 123, 125
Germany, 13–15, 19, 35–73, 140n. 2. *See also* MAKs
Grain dust, 86
Group size, 11–12, 68–69, 117

Halothane, 91
Health-based OELs, 20, 36–39, 105–7
Hematite, 138n. 3
Henschler, Dietrich, 36–37
Heptane, 126, 129
Heptanone, 137n. 9
Hexane, 50–51, 65, 93, 126, 129
Hexanone, 49–50, 53, 93
Hexylene glycol, 86
Högberg, Johan, 98
Holland, 19, 120
Holmberg, Bo, 95, 138n. 13
Homeopathy, 30
Hormones, 30
Hydrogen chloride, 129
Hydrogen cyanide, 129
Hydrogen fluoride, 86, 129
Hydrogen peroxide, 86

Hydrogen phosphide, 131
Hydrogen selenide, 129
Hydrogen sulfide, 30, 84, 129
Hydroquinone, 137n. 10
Hypothesis testing, 8

IBT (Industrial Bio-Test Laboratories), 32
India, 19
Indium, 94
Individual variation, 5, 20–21, 23, 43–45, 119
Indonesia, 19
Industrial Bio-Test Laboratories, 32
Industrial hygienists, 18, 28
Industrial Medical Association, 28
Information
 corporate, 27–29, 76
 to the public, 121
Interpolation, 139n. 10
Interpretation, toxicological, 110–13
Iodine, 30, 129
Ionizing radiation, 30, 125
Ireland, 19
Iron oxide, 126, 129
Irritation effects, 22, 39–43, 53, 82 88, 101, 135n. 4
Isoamyl alcohol, 129
Isocyanates, 29, 88, 90
Isophorone, 86, 126, 129
Isopropanol, 86, 129
Isopropyl ether, 130
Israel, 19
Italy, 32

Japan, 13–14, 19, 140n. 2

Keplinger, Moreno, 31–32
Kidney, 93–94

Index

Kramer, C.G., 31
Kreek, F.W. van der, 58, 136n. 7

Lead, 4, 45, 130
LEBEL, 115–17
Lefemine, G., 31
Leukemia, 11, 98
Levi, Isaac, 8
Linear extrapolation, 115–17
Liver, 83, 93
LOAEL, 43
Louis, Pierre Charles-Alexandre, 2
Lung cancer, 11

Magnesium oxide, 130
Magnuson, Harold, 20
MAKs, 35–73, 102, 106–7, 116–117
Malathion, 67
Malaysia, 19
Maleic anhydride, 61–62, 85
Malnutrition, 135n. 6
Maltoni, C., 31, 69–70
Manganese, 92–93, 130
Mastromatteo, Ernest, 22
Measurement technology, 26
Mechanistic knowledge, 6–7
Median value, 123
Medical values, 106, 108
Medicine, clinical, 1–3, 105
Mercury, 130
Mesityl oxide, 130
Metabolic rate, 112–13
Metabolism, 4–5, 68, 118
Metal fume fever, 95
Methanol, 130
Methoxyethanol, 54–55, 68, 130
Methoxyethyl acetate, 130
Methyl acetate, 86, 130
Methyl acrylate, 64

Methyl alcohol, 130
Methyl bromide, 92, 130
Methyl butanone, 126, 130
Methyl cellosolve, 130
Methyl cellosolve acetate, 130
Methyl chloride, 92, 130
Methyl chloroform, 92–93
Methylcyclohexane, 130
Methylcyclohexanol, 130
Methylcyclohexanone, 126, 130
Methylene chloride, 129
Methylene dianiline, 137n. 11
Methyl ethyl ketone, 93, 130
Methyl formate, 130, 137n. 8
Methyl isobutyl ketone, 130
Methyl isopropyl ketone, 130
Methyl mercaptan, 138n. 18
Methyl mercury, 46
Methyl methacrylate, 61–63, 86
Methyl pentanone, 130
Methyl propyl ketone, 131
Methyl pyrrolidone, 54, 56
Mexico, 19
Mineral fibers, 96
Minority opinions, 121–22
Monobromoethane, 129
Monochlorobenzene, 130
Monochloroethane, 129
Monochloromethane, 130
Monofluorotrichloromethane, 130
Mononitrotoluene, 130
Morpholine, 137n. 8
Morton, William, 19
Mutchler, T.E., 31

NAEL, 10
National Institute for Occupational Safety and Health, 19–20, 23
Negative list, 109
NEL, 10, 82

Netherlands, 19, 120
NIOSH, 19–20, 23
Nitrobenzene, 130
Nitroethane, 130
Nitrogen dioxide, 90, 126, 130
Nitrogen monoxide, 93, 137n. 10
Nitroglycerin, 130
Nitroglycol, 28
Nitromethane, 130, 137n. 8
Nitropropane, 86
Nitrotoluene, 126, 130
NOAEL, 10
NOEL, 10, 67–70, 114
Normal workers, 22, 44
Nose breathing, 59, 64–65
Numerical method, 2

OBEL, 115, 139n. 9
Occupational Health Program, 29
Occupational hygienists, 18, 28
Occupational medicine, 3–7, 9
Occupational Safety and Health Administration, 18–20, 72
Octane, 130
OELs. *See also* TLVs, MAKs
  ceiling values, 18, 86, 126–27
  default values, 108
  documentation, 14–15, 18, 24, 27, 35, 76, 81, 102, 110
  exception values, 108–9
  German, 35–73
  health-based, 20, 36–39, 105–7
  history, 12–13
  international comparisons, 13–15, 77–78
  medical values, 106, 108
  methods for comparing, 123–31
  reduction, 24–26, 38, 76–78
  residual values, 109–10

revision, 33, 72, 102
Swedish, 75–102
technological, 36–37
terminology, 133n. 1
time-weighted averages, 126–27
updating, 33, 72, 102
OHP, 29
Organogenesis, 46
OSHA, 18–20, 72
Ozone, 90, 130

Paper dust, 91
Parasitic diseases, 135n. 6
Parkinson's disease, 92
Pathology, 7
Peer review, 24, 26, 29, 34
Pentachloronaphthalene, 130
Pentane, 126, 131
Pentanol, 129
Pentanone, 126, 131
Perchloroethylene, 131
Peripheral nervous system, 93
Pesticides, 109–10
Philippines, 13–14, 19, 140n. 2
Phosgene, 131
Phosphine, 131
Phosphorous chloride, 131
Phosphorous trichloride, 131
Phthalic anhydride, 86–87
Piperazine, 89, 100–102
Pneumonia, 2
PNS, 93
Polyisocyanates, 90
Polyneuritis, 53
Polyneuropathy, 93
Polyvinyl chloride, 137n. 8
Portugal, 19
Positive list, 109
Pregnant workers, 45–47
Presumptions, 111

Index

Propyl acetate, 126, 131
Propylene glycol monomethyl ether, 86
Propylene oxide, 138n. 14
Pseudoscience, 30

Quartz, 28

Radiation, ionizing, 30, 125
Radon, 125
Reduction of OELs, 24–26, 38, 76–78
Regulations group, 76, 85, 98
Regulatory ratio, 48, 59, 82, 102, 136n. 6
Residual values, 109–10
Respiratory diseases, 82–83, 88–91
  lung cancer, 11
Revision of OELs, 33, 72, 102
Risk communication, 121
RR (regulatory ratio), 48, 59, 82, 102, 136n. 6
Russia, 13–14, 140n. 2. *See also* Soviet Union
Ruth, J.H., 101

Safety factor (uncertainty factor), 10, 20, 24, 46–49, 52–53, 58–59, 64, 73, 85, 104, 116, 136n. 6, 139n. 9. *See also* Regulatory ratio
  for effect vs. no-effect level, 64, 85
Salter, Liora, 20
Saturation, 118
Scaling factors, 112–13, 139
Schultz, William, 9
Science
  burden of proof, 8–11
  medical, 1–7
  role in standard-setting, 119–22
  separation from policy issues, 75–76, 102, 120–22
  and values, 104–5, 120–22
Selenium, 95, 99
Self-inflicting regulations, 105
Sex hormones, 30
Significance, statistical, 9–10, 113–14, 133n.3
Silver, 95
Smoking, 7, 11, 21, 23
Sodium fluoride, 126, 129
Solvents, 77
South Africa, 19
Soviet Union, 13, 15, 30. *See also* Russia
Spain, 19
Standard list, 124–31
Statistical significance, 9–10, 113–14, 133n. 3
Statistics
  confidence level, 139n. 9
  detection level, 113–14
  error types, 7–11, 113
  group size, 11–12, 68–69, 117
  history, 2–3
  hypothesis testing, 8
  significance, 9–10, 113–14, 133n. 3
Stibine, 131
Stokinger, Herbert, 21–23, 25, 28–33
Styrene, 92, 131
Subpopulations. *See* Individual differences
Substance level, 106–8
Sulfhydryl, 32–33
Sulfur chloride, 131
Sulfur dioxide, 38, 90, 131
Sulfuric acid, 131
Sulfur monochloride, 131
Surgeon General, 7

Index 165

Sweden, 13–15, 19, 75–102, 120, 124, 140n. 2
Switzerland, 19
2,4,5-T, 54, 58
Talc, 91
Teeth, 22
Tellurium, 131
Teratogenicity, 46, 94. *See also* Embryotoxicity
Terpenes, 90
tert-butylphenol, 50–51
Tetrachloroethane, 131
Tetrachloroethylene, 41, 131
Tetrachloromethane, 128
Tetra ethyl orthosilicate, 129
Tetryl, 126, 131
Thailand, 19
Thiram, 42, 138n. 16
Third World, 135n. 6
Thoron, 125
Thresholds, 30–33, 37, 116–17
Thyroid, 95
Time-weighted average, 126–27
Titanium dioxide, 91
TL, 82
TLVs, 17–34, 125–27, 136n. 8
  compared to Swedish OELs, 77
  corporate information, 27
  degree of protection, 20–26, 73
  documentation, 18, 24, 27
  economic considerations, 23
  harmful effects below, 24–26
  history, 17–19
  international influence, 19, 75, 135n. 6
  official use, 18–19
  reduction, 24–26
  revision, 33, 72
  success of, 20
  updating, 20
  used for air pollution standards, 20
  used to evaluate compensation claims, 19–20
TNT (*2,4,6*-trinitrotoluene), 38, 72, 126, 131
Toluene, 43, 131
Toluene diisocyanate, 25
Toluidine, 126, 131
Trace quantities, 30
Trichlorobenzene, 61, 63, 93, 137n. 11
Trichloroethane, 42
Trichloroethylene, 45, 50–51, 53, 70–71, 131
Trichlorofluoromethane, 53–54
Trichloromethane, 128
Trichloromonofluoromethane, 130
Trichloronaphthalene, 131
Trichlorotrifluoroethane, 60–61
Triethyl amine, 61, 63, 94
Trimellitic anhydride, 84
Trinitrophenylmethylnitramine, 131
Trinitrotoluene, 38, 72, 126, 131
TRK, 37
Tumors, 9, 11, 32, 36, 76–78, 96–98
Turkey, 13 14, 140n. 2
TWA, 126–27

Unborn children, 45–47, 94–95
Uncertainty factor. *See* safety factor
United Kingdom, 13–14, 19, 140n. 2
United States of America. *See also* TLVs
  offical OELs, 18–19
Updating, 33, 72, 102
Uranium, 28, 30
USSR, 13, 15, 30

Vanadium, 30, 90
Vanadium pentoxide, 28, 50–51, 53
van der Kreek, F.W., 58, 136n. 7
Venezuela, 19
Vinegar, 87
Vinyl acetate, 86–88, 135n. 4
Vinyl chloride, 4, 30–33, 118, 131
Vinylidene chloride, 31, 54, 56–57, 69–70
Vinyl toluene, 86
Volunteer exposures, 3, 22

Watanabe, P.G., 32
Wedeen, Richard, 24
White spirit, 86
WHO, 136n. 7
Wollastonite, 137n. 8
Women, 45–47
Work capacity, 42–43
Workers' compensation claims, 20
Workplace level, 106, 108
Work process level, 106, 108

Xylene, 71–72, 126, 131

Yugoslavia, 19

Zielhuis, R.L., 58, 136n. 7
Ziem, Grace, 24, 26
Zinc, 95
Zinc dimethyl dithiocarbamate, 138n. 14
Zinc oxide, 131